R.B. Abdullaev
A.M. Bakhtiyarova

ECOLOGICAL AND MEDICO-SOCIAL ASPECTS OF THE ARAL SEA PROBLEMS

R.B. Abdullaev
A.M. Bakhtiyarova

ECOLOGICAL AND MEDICO-SOCIAL ASPECTS OF THE ARAL SEA PROBLEMS

ScienciaScripts

Cover image: www.ingimage.com

This book is a translation from the original published under ISBN 978-620-7-64754-5.

Publisher:
Sciencia Scripts
is a trademark of
Dodo Books Indian Ocean Ltd. and OmniScriptum S.R.L publishing group

120 High Road, East Finchley, London, N2 9ED, United Kingdom
Str. Armeneasca 28/1, office 1, Chisinau MD-2012, Republic of Moldova, Europe
Managing Directors: Ieva Konstantinova, Victoria Ursu
info@omniscriptum.com

Printed at: see last page
ISBN: 978-620-8-57044-6

Contents

Compilers:
R.B.Abdullaev - Doctor of Medical Sciences, Professor, Department of Internal Medicine, Rehabilitation and Folk Medicine, Urgench Branch of Tashkent Medical Academy
A.M.Bakhtiyarova - student of the medical faculty of Urgench branch of the Tashkent Medical Academy
The book is devoted to the ecological crisis of the Aral Sea, ecological and economic consequences of this tragedy, health problems in the region of Southern Priaralie. The monograph contains completed and ongoing scientific research on the study of public health and development of measures for a new approach to the diagnosis, treatment and prevention of eco-dependent diseases. The monograph is dedicated to a wide range of readers, as well as ecologists, researchers, doctors and medical students.
Reviewers:
1. I.K. Abdullaev - Doctor of Medical Sciences, Professor, Head of the Department of Public Health and Health Management, Urgench Branch of the Tashkent Medical Academy
2. A.U.Ermekbaeva - Doctor of Medical Sciences, Professor, Head of the Department of Internal Medicine and Family Medicine, Karakalpak State Medical Institute

INTRODUCTION

Ecological problems represent a serious violation of the relationship between man and nature: it is the depletion of natural resources, violation of ecological balance, climate change, complications of living conditions and activities of people. The essence of ecological problems is that how reasonable, purposeful interrelations between man and nature.

Ecological security and environmental protection are the most important conditions for ensuring general, real national security, stable development and progress of society. The environmental problem has become one of the acute global problems of our time. Environmental problems, if they are not solved in time, can lead to disasters, loss of significant funds and time, complication of people's lives on the scale of one country, a separate region and the whole world.

General factors of anthropogenic impact on the environment (urbanisation, industrial and household waste, chemicalisation of everything and especially agriculture, air polluting transport, etc.) have many times aggravated consequences in the special conditions of Central Asia, such as the proximity of deserts, hot climate, the need for artificial irrigation of land, high population density in some areas, cotton monoculture, which depletes water resources.

One of the most dangerous zones of ecological disaster has developed in the Central Asian region. The processes of pollution of drinking water, atmosphere, reduction of sowing areas, etc. have not passed Uzbekistan. These processes have not passed Uzbekistan, where, according to experts, an extremely difficult, one can say, dangerous situation is developing:

1. The threat of limited land and its low quality composition.
2. Severe shortage and pollution of water resources.
3. The problem of the Aral Sea.
4. Air pollution.

The leadership of the Republic of Uzbekistan pays great attention to environmental protection and the rational use of natural resources. Legislative acts have been adopted and a number of international treaties and agreements have been concluded on the most important issues of environmental protection. The main areas of strengthening environmental security at present are:

1. Stopping pollution of air and water environment, by developing and implementing appropriate technology and strictly controlling the use of pesticides and other substances.
2. Rational use of all types of natural resources and ensuring natural expansion of reproduction of renewable resources and strictly calculated consumption of non-renewable ones.
3. Targeted, science-based transformation of natural conditions in large areas.
4. Preservation of the entire natural gene pool of wildlife as a source base, breeding new species of cultivated plants and animals.

5. Creating favourable living conditions for the population in cities and other settlements by maintaining a system of science-based urban planning and district planning.
6. Drawing the attention of the world community to the environmental problems of the region.

In his speech, the President of Uzbekistan paid special attention to the problem of climate change, stressing that today every country is feeling the devastating impact of this process.

"Unfortunately, these negative changes also pose a serious threat to the sustainable development of Central Asia. I would like to draw attention once again to the devastating consequences of the drying up of the Aral Sea. The Aral Sea area has become the epicentre of an environmental catastrophe," said the President of Uzbekistan.

"Emphasise the need for immediate action to restore the Aral Sea ecosystem, including improved water management and sustainable resource use."

"We call for the cooperation of all stakeholders, including states, international organisations and civil society, to achieve the common goal of preserving this unique natural resource."

The ecological catastrophe and socio-economic problems of the Aral Sea have aroused great interest from the scientific community and mass media in recent decades. The sea becomes a symbol of anthropogenic human interference in the natural environment and shows what can happen to water bodies under their intensive and insufficiently thought-out economic use. All this makes it necessary to carry out further studies of the inland water body.

The Aral Sea, a drainless salt lake in Central Asia, on the border of Kazakhstan and Uzbekistan, has for many decades made a great contribution to the economy of the former USSR, being one of the largest bodies of water rich in various species of flora and fauna. The Syr Darya and Amu Darya rivers supplied the sea with water and determined its volume, sea fish was exported, agriculture in the region was stimulated and provided with water. (N. O. Ignatyeva, 2022).

Salt and dust storms, which are blown from the bottom of the Aral Sea, pollute the Earth's atmosphere. Dust storms provoke the process of secondary desertification. Powerful jet atmospheric currents flowing from west to east carry aerosol mixtures of dust and salts from the Aral Sea bed to the surface of glaciers of the Tien Shan and Pamir. Pollution of glaciers intensifies the already active melting caused by global climate change. Glaciers are the treasure trove of fresh water reserves for the countries of Central Asia and therefore the melting process is very dangerous for these countries. It is necessary to develop a management strategy and mechanisms to coordinate the use of water basins. Despite the catastrophic situation of the Aral Sea, water is still seen in Central Asian countries as an energy and water resource.

irrigation resource. The consequence of this is the deterioration of drinking water quality, which affects the health of the population, the amount of fertile and productive land is decreasing, the quality of life is deteriorating, poverty and unemployment are increasing, and migration rates are high. United efforts of all countries will give an opportunity to implement joint projects on saving the Aral Sea for the welfare of the future generation. (G.S.Tileukulova, 2022).

Taking into account the crucial role of ecology in the life of the population of the Central Asian countries, the heads of these five states gathered in 1993 in Kazakhstan and having discussed the emerging environmental situation adopted a joint agreement on joint actions to prevent the drying up of the Aral Sea and its consequences. To solve the set tasks, the Heads of State decided to establish the Interstate Council on the Aral Sea Problems and its working body - the Executive Committee. The International Fund for Saving the Aral Sea has been established for financial support of the above tasks. The second meeting of the Supreme Heads of the Central Asian republics was held in Nukus in 1994. Here the "Programme of concrete actions on improvement of ecological situation in the Aral Sea basin for the next thirty years taking into account the socio-economic development of the region" was approved. In the same year in Dashkhauz of the Republic of Turkmenistan the report of the Interstate Council on the implementation of this programme was heard.

Governments of the Central Asian republics, international organisations adopted on 20 September 1995 in Nukus of the Republic of Uzbekistan the Declaration of the Central Asian states and international organisations on the problems of sustainable development of the Aral Sea region. This declaration envisages solution of such crucial problems as:

— transition to a more balanced and science-based system of agriculture and forestry;

Improving the efficiency of irrigation through the development of economic methods of water resources use, application of advanced technologies in irrigation and environmental protection;

— Improvement of the system of integrated management of natural resources in the region.

In 1997 in Almaty a regular meeting of the Heads of five Central Asian states with participation of the UN and World Bank representatives was held, where a decision was made to improve organisational structures for solving the Aral Sea problems - a more efficient composition of the International Fund for Saving the Aral Sea was formed.

According to the Resolution of the President of the Republic of Uzbekistan No. F-4330 dated 5 August 2014 "An international conference on the implementation of regional projects in the Aral Sea basin was held in Urgench"

Decree of the Cabinet of Ministers No. 1031 dated 24.12.2019 on the creation of "green covers" in the arid areas of the Aral Sea was adopted.

On the initiative of the leader of our country, 500 thousand hectares of green areas (shrubs) are being created this year to stop desertification caused by the construction of the Aral Sea.

PART 1

ENVIRONMENTAL CRISIS IN THE ARAL SEA AREA

The negative consequences of the environmental catastrophe in the Aral Sea region go far beyond just the regions, becoming planetary in nature. Thus, millions of tonnes of caustic dust blown up by winds from the dried-up sea bed are already falling as salty rain in a number of regions of the Russian Federation, Belarus, Lithuania and other even more remote places. All this shows that delay in eliminating the crisis situation that has developed here may lead to more serious moral and economic costs. Therefore, in-depth study of the ecological, sanitary-epidemiological situation and development of comprehensive recommendations on health protection and restoration of the natural environment in the Aral Sea region is one of the urgent scientific and practical tasks.

Nature and society are a single dynamic system and changes in the biosphere cannot but affect the biological nature of man. Deterioration of the ecological situation immediately affects the health of the population living in the zone of ecological disadvantage. The further improvement of living conditions of the present and future generation of people depends to a large extent on environmental factors. Over the last 15-20 years, the Republic of Uzbekistan has faced the problem of sharp deterioration of the environment and natural resources. Especially the drying up of the Aral Sea has been a real ecological disaster. This is not only an ecological, but also an economic, medical and demographic disaster in the Aral Sea region, affecting the fate of the peoples of Uzbekistan, Kazakhstan and Turkmenistan.

Environmental factors influencing the crisis in the Aral Sea and its adjacent Aral Sea area

Sea and its adjacent territory of Priaralie

"The Blue Eye of the Earth" - the Aral Sea emerged more than 35,000 years ago.

It is the largest lake in Central Asia. It has an area of 66,458 kilometres square (with islands). It was the fourth largest in the world (after the Caspian Sea, Lake Superior in America and Lake Victoria in Africa). The greatest length was from north-east to south-west 428 km, width at 450 north latitude 284 km. The Aral Sea has no drainage.

The Aral Sea embraces two huge rivers, the Amu Darya and the Syr Darya. The northern shores of the Aral Sea, in some places low-lying, are cut by large bays; the northern shores are adjoined by the sands of the Great Badgers, the Small Badgers and the Priaralie Karakums. The eastern shores are low-lying, sandy, strongly heated with many small bays and sandy islands. The southern bank is formed by the huge Amu Darya delta. The western shore is precipitous, in some places rising 190 metres above the level of the Aral Sea, devoid of bays, and represents the eastern edge of the Ust-Yurt plateau. Of the islands (total area of islands-2.345 km sq. km) the largest are: Kugaral (area 273 km sq. km), Vozrozhdeniya (216 km sq. km), Barsa-Kelmes ("you go - you will not return", 133 km), near the delta Amu Darya - Tokmak - Ata. In the north - the eastern tip of the Aral Sea railway station "Aral Sea".

As a result of the decrease in the level of the Aral Sea by more than 40.42 metres, it is no longer a single sea, but two residual lakes. Its shores have retreated over 70-110 kilometres. The deltas of the Amu Darya and Syr Darya are intensively degrading. Bottom desiccation was found on the area of more than 4 million hectares. In return, we have received another man-made sandy-solonchak desert. The winds from the dried Aral Sea bed lift salt and dust into the air and carry them hundreds of kilometres away.

In the recent past - in the 50s, the height of the Aral Sea was 53 metres, its area was almost 67 thousand square kilometres, its water volume was 1062 cubic metres, and its salinity was 10 g/l. The Amu Darya and Syr Darya annually poured 60 cubic metres of water into the sea. This constituted 81% of the total incoming part of the water balance, the remaining part was accounted for by groundwater and rainwater.

Since 1960, the water level started to decrease, with an average annual decrease of 0.21 metres between 1961 and 1970, 0.58 metres between 1971 and 1980, and 1.0 metres since 1980. By 1990, the water level had dropped by 14 metres compared to 1960, the total sea area had decreased by 40%, the water volume by 60%, and the average salinity had reached 30 t/l. In 1982, 1986 the rivers did not inject water into the sea at all, and since 1981 navigation in the sea has completely stopped. The main reasons for this tragedy are: firstly, constant increase of irrigated lands (over 3 million hectares of land have been developed in the Aral Sea region over the last 35 years); secondly, construction of large irrigation facilities (over 50 reservoirs have been built in Central Asia).

By 1994, the water level in the Aral Sea had dropped to 32.5 m, the volume was less than 400 cubic kilometres, and the mirror area was 8032.5 thousand square kilometres. water mineralisation had doubled.

Dust storms on the dried bottom of the Aral Sea were first detected as a result of space research back in 1975. Since the 1980s, such storms have been observed here for 90 days a year. Dust plumes reach 400 kilometres in length and 40 kilometres in width, and the radius of action of dust storms is up to 300 kilometres. According to experts' estimates, between 15 and 75 million tonnes of dust rise into the atmosphere here every year.

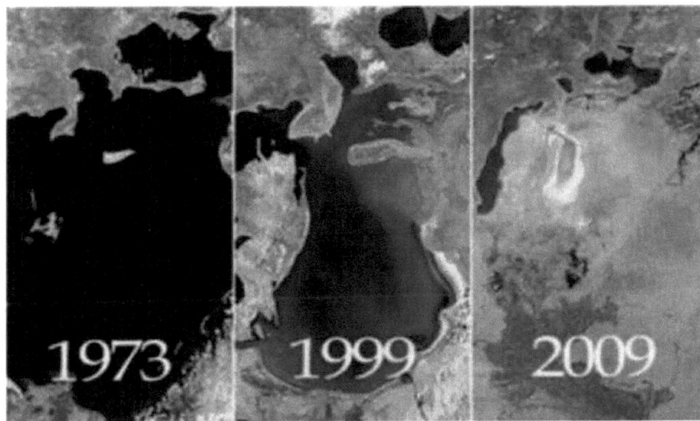

Fig. View from space. The Aral Sea in 1973,1999,2009.

Since 1983, the Aral Sea has ceased to exist as a place of fish production. Far from the modern coastline one can find rusty islands of once powerful fishing fleet, ruined settlements of fishermen. Bozkol, Altynkol, Karatma bays disappeared, Akpetki archipelago merged with the land. Pastures and hayfields are disappearing, territories are swamping. Growing water deficit and deteriorating water quality caused degradation of soils and vegetation cover, changes in flora and fauna, as well as reduction of irrigated agriculture efficiency.

The Aral Sea tragedy is, in fact, a global environmental catastrophe. The collisions in the interaction between society and nature that have arisen in the Aral Sea region, reflecting on the conditions of human existence, socio-economic processes of the present, affect the health of people living here, determine the main content of the environmental problem. On foreign ecological maps this region is labelled as the triangle of death. This region is also called "silent Chernobyl" (Berdimuratova A., 1997). The unheard-of grief did not suddenly fall on it, but slowly crept in, destroying people's health.

The threatening environmental situation every year claims many human lives and increases the number of dangerous diseases. The lives of hundreds of thousands of people living in this territory are at risk.

The most negative consequences take place in the Southern Priaralie (Table 1). While the total area of the Aral Sea region is 473 thousand square kilometres, the area of its southern part is 245 thousand square kilometres or 19.2% of the territory of Central Asia. This includes the entire territory of the Republic of Karakalpakstan, Khorezm vilayat and Tashauz province of Turkmenistan. The ongoing ecological disturbances, and by the example of the Aral Sea and Priaralie in terms of intensity of desertification processes have no analogues in the world practice, this explains the difficulties of quantitative and qualitative assessment of ecological changes. Today more than 10 million people live in the zone of ecological disaster (Zhirinkov G.A., 1993).

Ecological changes in the region are inextricably linked to the fate of the Syr Darya and Amu Darya rivers, which, together with the glaciers that feed them and the Aral Sea itself, form a single complex created by nature itself: mountains - rivers - sea. However, as a result of extensive management and wasteful use of water resources, the existing natural balance has been artificially disturbed, as a result of which a vast arid zone has emerged in the lower reaches of the Syr Darya, especially in the Aral Sea area, where up to 0.5 million inhabitants of the Kzyl-Orda region live. The unprecedented 28-year reduction of river water inflow into the sea has led to a 14-metre drop in its level and a 65% drop in water volume, and its salinity has increased from 11-12 to 26-27 g/litre. Only within Kazakhstan the sea bottom has been exposed on the area of 1.3, and in general - more than 2.5 million hectares. Its warm humid breath now does not protect it from the scalding effect of desert winds, on the contrary, a new dust and salt centre with sand dunes and sparse solanaceous vegetation was formed on the vast dried seabed. The radius of its influence includes a wide range of settlements in the Aral and Kazaly districts, including the Aral itself (Kulmanov M.E., 1996).

One of the reasons for the Aral Sea's death is insufficient water inflow from the two rivers Amu Darya and Syr Darya, so if in 1960 the Aral Sea received 58.8 cubic kilometres of water per year, in 1989 it dropped to 4.3 cubic kilometres.

Total water inflow from the Amu Darya and Syr Darya averaged 42.9 cubic kilometres in 1960-1971, 16.1 cubic kilometres in 1971-1980, and only 4.3 cubic kilometres in 1981-1984. Since 1978, water inflow from the Syr Darya has stopped and from the Amu Darya has decreased to 1-5 cubic kilometres per year.

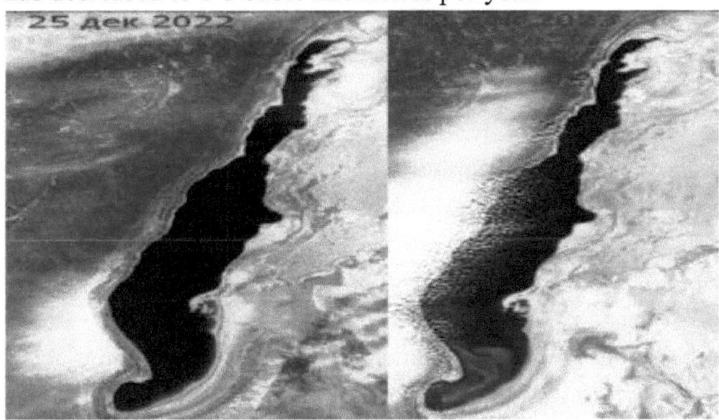

Fig. Aral Sea 25 December 2022 and 12 December 2023 view from the Aral Sea of space.

The use of Amu Darya water for irrigation, land reclamation and irrigation has significantly changed the ecosystem of the Khorezm Vilayat region. Reduction of water flow in rivers led to decrease of alluvial component, microorganisms feeding soil, depletion of groundwater reserves, as a result of which water from the channel was absorbed into soil and groundwater level along the Amudarya river bank dropped by 6-8 metres, causing salinisation of coastal soil, change of flora along the bank.

The soil of the Amudarya delta, previously belonging to the hydromorphological or poly morphological complex, is becoming more arid and saline. Salt content in the soil reaches 30%, and saline layers are found at the depth of 1.5-2.0 metres.

Expansion of irrigation systems network, development of new lands, water use for industrial and economic needs reduced water flow rate in the Amu Darya River on the one hand, and on the other hand, low efficiency of water use, mismanagement, wastage, lack of appropriate drainage systems, high degree of soil salinity for washing of water used for irrigation resulted in excessive salinity of water in the upper reaches of the river, which then flows to the region of Khorezm.

Thus, for the last decades seasonal salinisation of water in the lower reaches of the Amu Darya River in Khorezm Vilayat has increased 2-4 times, sometimes reaching the level of 2.1-2.2 grams per litre, and in some low-water periods up to 3.0 grams per litre.

Highly mineralised water and saline soil have a detrimental effect on agricultural production. Losses in agriculture are growing annually, which affect the whole economy of Khorezm Vilayat, as insignificant degree of soil salinity causes 20.0% decrease in crop yields, and high salt content - 50.0%.

Another reason for the aggravation of the ecological crisis is the ecological and socio-cultural contradictions that determine the relationship between each stage of the historical development of man and nature. Therefore, the first condition for radical change of the current situation is a clear realisation that it is impossible to create a powerful economy without solving the ecological problem in a cardinal way, as there can be no healthy economy with a "sick ecology". In this regard, we need to solve the following problems: firstly, to develop a philosophical foundation for a new global ecological consciousness. The ideas of universal spiritual unity, the sacredness of each human life and humanity as a single family, the well-being of all members of society provide the basis for global environmental consciousness.

Secondly, in the conditions of transition to market relations with the help of the political system, mass media to spread these ideas, to make them a necessary part of human thinking. Therefore, the most important point of application of efforts for the normalisation of the ecological situation is the rule of law, an effective economic mechanism that stimulates entrepreneurship to the maximum extent possible, consolidation of the priority of needs of the individual, ensuring human rights.

Thirdly, taking into account the fact that one of the main criteria of progressiveness of socio-economic system is the ability of society to use the achievements of scientific and technical progress with minimum damage to the environment, the largest factor of socio-economic progress of the present time - scientific and technical progress - will be involved in our republic.

Further causes of the worsening ecological crisis include the spontaneous or insufficiently conscious appropriation of nature's riches by humanity and the dynamics of demographic factors. The core of the demographic factor is a continuously reproducing population of people, i.e. the population. The development of society and nature depends on such demographic indicators as total population size, growth rate, sex and age structure, state of psychophysical health, and migration mobility. What effect migration has in a particular case depends on its rate, direction and structure of migration flows. In the Aral Sea region migration is a consequence of the ecological crisis. According to the Ministry of Economic Statistics of the Republic of Karakalpakstan, in 1996, 6500 people left rural areas, and in subsequent years this figure has been gradually increasing. The migration flow is mainly dominated by the

15

Young people are the most able-bodied and educated part of the population.

Environmental and economic consequences environmental disaster

Khorezm Vilayat is located in the north-western part of the Republic of Uzbekistan, in

the lower reaches of the Amu Darya River, on its left bank, three hundred kilometres from the coast of the Aral Sea. The environmental, economic and social situation in the Aral Sea region, including the Khorezm Vilayat, is difficult. In the North, the vilayat borders with the Republic of Karakalpakstan (Amu Darya fog). In the North-East its border is the Amu Darya River, on the right bank of the river are located Beruni and Turtkul fogs of the Republic of Karakalpakstan. In the West and in the South Vilayat borders with Tashauz and Darganata provinces of the Republic of Turkmenistan. Vilayat was formed on 15 January 1938. The territory of Vilayat is 813, 9 thousand square kilometres. The region is divided into 11 administrative tumans and two cities Urgench, Khiva. The population of vilayat as of 01.01.2000 is 1,314,621 people. The centre of the vilayat is the city of Urgench with a population of 146,721. The climate of Khorezm Vilayat is sharply continental. The average annual air temperature is +11 +13 degrees Celsius, the hottest month is July, the average temperature of which is + 30 degrees Celsius, and in some days reaches 45 degrees Celsius, the coldest month is January with the average monthly air temperature of -6 -9 degrees Celsius and the maximum -27 degrees Celsius. The multi-year average annual rainfall is60 - 120 mm. The greatest amount of precipitation falls on autumn-spring months. Characteristic for Vilayat are constantly blowing winds - in autumn, winter and spring - of the North-Eastern direction, in summer - of the Northern direction. Their average annual speeds reach 2.1-4.8 m/sec, maximum (in spring) winds can reach 10-15 m/sec, minimum in autumn - 1.8-2.2 m/sec. Proximity of Karakum deserts
16
and Kyzylkum with high summer air temperatures and constantly blowing winds affect humidity in Khorezm Vilayat. The average annual humidity does not exceed 55-60%, relative humidity in winter is 70-80%, in summer it drops to 33-54%.

In Vilayat, a wide network of irrigation canals, close groundwater table, increased soil moisture, high solar radiation causes increased evaporation of moisture. The highest value of moisture evaporation is observed from May to August, reaching 350 mm, the lowest in December-January.

Geomorphologically, the lands of Khorezm are alluvial deposits, represented by sands, loams and clays of the fourth age. Rich in alluvial components, lime, phosphate and microorganisms, the land is ideal for agriculture.

Relief of the vilayat is calm, flat. Ground frost depth is 0.8 metres. The hydrogeological network of the vilayat is represented by the Amu Darya River, branched irrigation and collector-drainage network, lakes. Groundwater is formed by filtration of surface water bodies. The minimum position of groundwater level is observed in December-April, maximum rise in June-August, long-term seasonal fluctuation of groundwater level is from 0.3 to 1.1 metres. Groundwater is highly corrosive to concrete and metals, its water is highly mineralised.

Vilayat is agro-industrial, the main branches of agriculture are cotton growing, grain growing, melon growing and cattle breeding. Among the industrial enterprises the largest are "Urgench-6" in Urgench city, carpet combine in Khiva city, "Gurlene -

textile" in Gurlene fog, cotton-processing enterprises.

The ecological crisis in Vilayat is a consequence of a major ecological catastrophe that befell this region (due to the shoaling of the Aral Sea). The main ways of solving the problem and getting out of the situation that arose here should be considered in the interrelation with the peculiarities of the whole region of the Aral Sea basin, its geographical and natural characteristics, in the dynamics of socio-economic and ecological development trends. The structure of cotton farming, which has developed over the last decade, did not allow to effectively solve socio-economic and ecological problems. Extensive development of irrigated farming, low level of agriculture and insufficient industrialisation under high rates of population growth and water resources use did not give the planned increase of average per capita income and level of life.

Such miscalculations were the result of the former "all-union" economic policy of farming aimed only at cotton production and export, which led to increased imbalance in the economy.

The problem of supplying the population with many necessary types of consumer goods remains acute. The Khorezm vilayat together with the Republic of Karakalpakstan occupies one of the last places in the Republic in terms of basic indicators of people's well-being, in particular average per capita income, provision of drinking water, sewerage, equipment of health care, public education and cultural institutions.

The low level of average per capita income in the Aral Sea region severely limits the possibilities of consumption and capital accumulation, as a result of which labour productivity has fallen, incomes in the production and non-production spheres of the economy have decreased, and due to untimely implementation of a set of environmental protection measures, the quantity and quality of drinking water and foodstuffs have decreased, the environment has changed, the living standards of the population have deteriorated, and the relatively high population growth of the region quickly absorbs the income of the industrial sector. As a result, the possibility of escaping the vicious circle of the region's ecological disaster with domestic resources is nullified. The combined effects of harsh living conditions, continued environmental degradation and economic reconstruction on the local population are only now being quantified.

Climate and soil changes

The climate of Khorezm Vilayat was mainly formed under the influence of the Aral Sea, but due to the crisis of the Aral Sea, the climate of Vilayat has changed, so the summer became hotter, drier, the air temperature in some months reached +50 degrees Celsius, winter became colder, the temperature mark fell and decreased to 30 - 40 degrees, also the amount of precipitation decreased to 80-100 mm. The number of windy days increased, thereby increasing the tendency of the Vilayat climate to move towards continental.

Along with land degradation, deterioration of drinking water quality, deterioration of living conditions of the population and other consequences, the climate of this region is changing dramatically. Sharp cooling, late onset of spring, constant cold, dusty winds are signs of recent years only, as the Aral Sea has been protecting Central Asia from cold northern winds for thousands of years. When meeting with a powerful column of vapours from its surface, cold air masses were thrown by "atmospheric lift" to the highest height, overcame the way of thousands of kilometres, filled the reserves of eternal snow of Pamir.

Sand and salt storms carrying thousands of tonnes of dust and salt from the shores of the Aral Sea reach Khorezm, polluting its air basin, soil and water, thus damaging the ecology and economy of the region.

According to experts, the drying of the Aral Sea affects the atmospheric circulation. The repetition of meridional durm in the atmospheric circulation (December-February) has especially intensified. Attention is drawn to the fact that the mineral composition of precipitation has changed. For example, according to the data of the weather station "Aral Sea" for 1969-1979, a sixfold 19

increase of minerals in atmospheric precipitation, this process especially increased 1974-1980 reaching a total mineralisation per year of 9.8 and 13.1 mg/l, with an increase in sulphate ions.

Comparisons of air temperature measurements for the years 1960-1979 show that large changes have occurred in the last ten years (1970-1979). This case is characteristic not only around the coast but also other meteorological stations far from the sea, such as Tomdi, Chunkozgon, Kulkuduk. Increase of continentality of climate is noted in Priaralie, daily air temperature fluctuation changes (Table 2).

It should be noted that if 1950-1959 in Muynak individual non-sedimentary days were 30-35 days during the year, then in 1970-1979 this indicator was 120-150 days (Alibekov L., 1994).

Irrigated land increased in the world since 1950s up to 3 more per cent per year, and the use of mineral fertilisers, pesticides increased up to 9 times. At the same time, food production of meat, grain, fish, rice and others increased by 3-6 times. However, extensive expansion of agrochemicals, violation of agrotechnical requirements without taking into account long-term consequences of such development led to the development of erosion processes, waterlogging and salinisation of lands, pollution of surface and underground water, decline in land fertility and crop yields, deterioration of ecological situation, reduction of species diversity of flora and fauna. By 1980-1985 the growth of irrigated lands in the world practically stopped, their degradation and withdrawal from turnover increased.

These processes and tendencies were typical for Central Asian republics, where irrigated lands increased at higher rates up to 5-10% per year and were planned by central authorities, under obvious deficit of water resources. This caused drying up of the Aral Sea and development of desertification on huge areas. All works on transferring part of the Siberian rivers' flow, surveys and designs were interrupted and frozen. Earlier in the region irrigated lands were concentrated in oases, floodplains, river deltas on 20 relatively light, non-saline and slightly saline soils and their use was based on thousands of years of rich experience and traditions of local population, economical use of water resources and organic fertilisers. After large-scale land development works in Hungry Degree, where perfect irrigation network was created - lined canals, flumes, closed drainage and ahead of construction of main diversion collectors, widespread development of more saline, difficult to reclaim lands started. These processes were extended to the lower reaches of the Amu Darya and Syr Darya rivers. Since 1970s, mass construction of collector-drainage network, development of new lands under rice and cotton growing, reconstruction of part of old irrigated lands was started. Unfortunately, the experience of Golodnaya and Karitinskaya degree development was transferred to the lower reaches of the Amudarya river, where weak natural drainability, insignificant land slopes, floating fine-sandy soils, and positive data on horizontal and vertical drainage operation are absent (Goldstein R., 1996).

Irrigated agriculture is of serious concern in the region: in the middle and lower parts of the Amu Darya and Syr Darya rivers, where saline lands prevail. 30-40 years practice of exploitation and reclamation, old and new irrigation systems leads to increasing mobilisation of salts from deep geological saline strata and their involvement in hydrochemical cycles, contributing to the growth of land salinisation. Increase of land drainability by means of specific drainage network did not give tangible results. Thus, in Khorezm vilayat, up to 1300 tonnes of salts were extracted from 1 ha of land over 35 years. At the same time in Karakalpakstan and Khorezm now there are practically no non-saline lands left, the area of medium and highly saline lands has increased up to 45-60%. At the same time, there is a continuous decline in cotton yield from 32-42 centners/ha to 18-30 centners/ha. The existing irrational system of furrow irrigation, earthen canal beds, leaching irrigation lead to large water losses for filtration, waterlogging and waterlogging of lands. This, in turn, causes anaerobic processes in the soil, which lead to changes in PH of the environment, release of toxic methane, carbon dioxide, extraction of metals bound in the soil: iron, aluminium, manganese and others. Mapping revealed significant salinisation of soil horizon in irrigated areas, caused not only by dust and salt emissions from the dried part of the Aral Sea, but also by intensive salinisation and evaporation. As a result of unregulated irrigation regime, about 50 per cent of lands in Khorezm Vilayat and 30 per cent in the Republic of Karakalpakstan were waterlogged. Groundwater level increased by 2-3 metres and more. In the general balance of saline lands prevail moderately saline and highly saline. Very highly saline lands (50 g/l and more) account for about 15% of the irrigated area (Goldstein R., 1996).

In addition to widespread soil salinisation, the works carried out have reliably established that about 40% of soils on the territory of Khorezm Vilayat are contaminated with such herbicides as DDG and HCCH, the amount of which reaches 17 MPC. Detailed works on separate contaminated sites, where after a year the concentration of pesticides was repeatedly determined, showed that the degree of contamination has not decreased, which proves that their use continues despite the ban.

In addition to pesticides, according to atmogeochemical survey data, soils and soils of the Aral Sea region are intensively polluted with fuel fractions of petroleum products. Foci of pollution are confined to urban agglomerations and are trickling along canals and collectors draining groundwater. Hydrocarbon pollution is most strongly manifested in Khorezm Vilayat.

The sown area of Khorezm Vilayat in 1998 was 235.9 thousand hectares, including 112.6 thousand hectares of cotton and 42.4 thousand hectares of grain crops.

The production of cotton, rice and other crops requires large quantities of water. A wide network of irrigation systems of crops requires large amounts of water. This network has aggravated the problem of soil salinisation; an intensive paradox is observed - highly mineralised water of irrigation systems secondary salinisation of soil. In the oblast more than 25% of arable land is soil with high salt content, Taking into account the fact that more than 15% of irrigated land is annually sown with rice, the main water consumer, the probability of salinisation and land turnover out of sowing is increasing. Changes in the structure and composition of soil have affected the fertility of land, annually on 5 thousand hectares of land in the region fertility decreases, there is an increase in soil eroded, the agrochemical structure of soil changes, the harvest of agricultural crops decreases.

Due to increase of water salinity, groundwater rise, ameliorative condition of lands has deteriorated, which annually leads to death of fruit-bearing orchards and vineyards. At present, more than all fruit-bearing orchards, grapes and mulberries are in thinned condition. In recent years, the use of mineral fertilisers and pesticides in agriculture has been decreasing, but their mismanagement in previous years has led to significant soil contamination, as every year pesticides are found in larger soil samples.

Salt dust carried by sandstorms from the Aral Sea water area and highly mineralised water from the Amu Darya River leads to changes in the core chemical and biological structure of the soil. This adversely affects agricultural productivity, flora and fauna of the environment and human health.

It is necessary to take into account the fact that unfavourable sanitary and ecological situation in the vilayat is formed on sanitary cleaning, improvement and sewerage of settlements. Annually more than 40 per cent of the established norms are removed solid waste from settlements, the rest remains in settlements polluting the soil with inorganic and organic substances. In rural settlements solid and liquid wastes are disposed of near residential houses, water bodies and on wastelands. In rural settlements there is no sewerage system, they use primitive backyard toilets and pit latrines, the effluents of which are absorbed by the soil and thus pollute the soil and subsoil groundwater with biological and chemical substances.

Soil contamination and salinity, high groundwater conditions, and extensive chemicalisation of agriculture have led to significant biological and chemical contamination of soil, which has manifested itself in changes in its morphological structure and microflora.

Various organic fertilisers and means of chemical protection of plants are widely used in vilayat to increase fertility and yield of agriculture. Thus, in 1993, 79117 tonnes of mineral fertilisers (for comparison, in 1992 - 71298 tonnes) and674, 7 tonnes of pesticides (in 1992 - 283,8 tonnes) were used in agriculture, while the consumption of pesticides per 1 ha of area was 5,4 kg (in 1992 - 2,02 kg) per capita - 0,5 kg (in 1992 - 0,24 kg). Although in 1994 the use of mineral fertilisers was reduced to 61395 tonnes and pesticides to 426.5 tonnes, the probability of environmental pollution is not reduced at all. In 1999, 40.3 per cent of water samples, 53.8 per cent of soil samples, 55.5 per cent of air samples during defoliation and 56.7 per cent of foodstuffs were found to contain pesticide residues. In 2000, pesticide residues were also detected in water samples, soil samples, atmospheric air samples and foodstuff samples, which did not significantly decrease in comparison with 1999.

Changes in water supply and composition

In Uzbekistan, the population coverage with centralised water supply is 75% in urban areas and 50% in rural areas. In the lower reaches of the Amu Darya river the population coverage with water supply does not exceed 65%, and in rural areas 10-20%. Survey of efficiency of purification and disinfection devices, monitoring of drinking water supply sources in the lower reaches of rivers, analysis of water quality by 30-40 pollution ingredients showed:

— high pollution of river waters, surface sources and failure of underground, canal and riverine lenses, due to increase of their mineralisation, high hardness, contamination with toxic organic, bacterial substances, agrochemicals, etc.;

— with distance from the river there is an increase in pollution of surface water, distributed through the canals up to 1.5-2.0 times for all components, especially in low-water years, in the period of autumn-spring land flushing;

Many settlements have primitive treatment facilities - settling tanks, sometimes quick sand filters and subsequent chlorination, without automatic devices for reagent supply. In this case, complex toxic organochlorine compounds (trihalomethane, etc.) are formed in drinking water;

— sanitary-parasitological studies of tap and well water samples, carried out for the first time together with the "Mycology" centre in Nukus city, Muynak, Takhiatash, Kungirad, showed the presence of helminths pathogenic for humans - eggs of ascarids, pinworms, cysts of non-pathogenic intestinal protozoa and pathogenic giardia resistant to chlorine doses. These pathogenic microorganisms were not detected only in tap water of Khojeyli city;

— practically no organisation carries out a complete comprehensive analysis of drinking water quality taking into account regional specificity of . The existing GOST "Drinking Water" does not take into account the low standard of living of the population, stresses from industrial pollution, use of high doses of agrochemicals, hot climate of the region and intake of large drinking water norms and others;

- There is no monitoring and mapping of pollution of the main sources of drinking water, no forecast of the intensity of pollution of underground sources of drinking

water, including the foothill zone of the region.
A similar analysis of drinking water in Tashauz province revealed non-compliance of the water used with GOST "Drinking water" in 60% of samples taken for analysis, and in the city of Tashauz 40%, and in a number of districts this value reaches 80% (Razzakov R.M., 1996).
It should be noted that for many years in the Aral Sea region huge doses of globally banned pesticides (DDT, hexachloran, butifos, propanil and others), as well as mineral fertilisers, the effect of which on the human body is poorly understood, were used. In addition, water from 146 collector systems was discharged into the Syr Darya from rice and cotton fields. And 114 of them were located outside the Kzil-Orda region of Kazakhstan. The mass of harmful substances getting into the sea, settle on the bottom.
In recent years, not only the hydrological regime of the Syr Darya has changed significantly, but also the physical and chemical composition of its water. Thus, from 1956 to 1989, its mineralisation at Kzyl-Orda increased by 3.4 times, and its chloride and sulphate content by 5.2 times. The value of total acidity increased from 0.05 to 0.7; nitrite - from 1.0 to 10.0 and acidity - from 3.0 to 7.0 mg/litre. It systematically detects pesticides, phenols, petroleum products, heavy metal salts and other components of industrial and agricultural effluents.
According to I.A.Usmanov (1996), anthropotechnogenic pressure on the environment, including the hydrosphere, leads to inhibition of bacteriological self-purification processes and, as a consequence, to increased bacterial contamination of water. This is clearly evidenced by the given data.
Dysentery, typhoid fever, typhoid 26
typhoid, salmonellosis, cholera and others. Meanwhile, the population of Kzyl-Orda, Kazalinsk, Tasbuget, Karmakcha, Novokazalinsk and others continue to partially use Syr-Darya water for household and drinking purposes due to the shortage of good quality drinking water.
It is necessary to pay attention to the fact that according to the data of Kulmanov M.E. and co-authors (1996) the intensive rates of the Aral Sea shoaling promoted and strengthening of processes of continental salinisation of underground waters, especially in the Aral and Kazalinsk districts, where the level of their mineralisation is 2300-3700 mg, so in 1995 it was predicted 5000-7000 mg/l and this forecast more than justified itself. As it is known, the degree of water hardness has a certain influence on the activity of the urinary system organs, the development of iron deficiency in the body, as well as cardiovascular and kidney stone diseases. Nevertheless, a significant part of the population of the above-mentioned districts continues to use well water. To date, only 67% of the population of Kzyl-Orda province is provided with centralised water supply. At the same time, the quality of water supplied in 21.5 per cent of cases does not meet GOST requirements in terms of bacterial indicator, and in 49 per cent of cases it is not harmful in terms of chemical composition. About 10% of residents use imported water and 4% use open water reservoirs.
It should be noted that despite the poor quality of drinking water, the availability of

water remains low. Thus, one rural inhabitant of the oblast receives on average 10-15 litres, and in district centres 17-25, in Kzyl-Orda 80 litres per day, which is 5-6 times lower than the norm. Until now, the problem of providing the population with quality drinking water is one of the priority problems requiring urgent solution. With the total water intake capacity of 128 thousand metres per day, only 45 thousand metres per day or 35% is supplied to the population, the rest of the water is used for production purposes. The situation is aggravated by the fact that out of 438 kilometres of water supply networks 196 (44.7) are in emergency condition, and a significant number of water intakes are not functioning. Water supply and sewerage facilities in Kzyl-Orda are in critical sanitary and technical condition (Kulmanov M.E., 1993).

In Uzbekistan, work has begun on the "Geoecology of Uzbekistan" programme, aimed at assessing the ecological state of all natural environments, identifying a wide range of pollutant elements and developing environmental protection measures. Geo-ecological studies and mapping of the Aral Sea region have been completed in the course of the programme. They have shown that the most negative factor causing the emergency situation in all districts of Uzbekistan, Kazakhstan and Turkmenistan, which are part of the Aral Sea region, is the poor quality of surface and ground waters. The two main water arteries - Amu Darya Syr Darya - are polluted with oil products, heavy metals and especially phenols (up to 10-20 MPC). Groundwater is saline throughout the territory, and in some areas is still polluted with phenols, pesticides and oil products. The lenses of fresh water used for drinking water supply that existed along the main canals are gradually mineralising. Of the 37 freshwater lenses explored in Karakalpakstan, only 12 are currently exploited, and those with water mineralisation 1-1.8 g/l. The Khorezm Vilayat and the Republic of Karakalpakstan are completely deprived of water supply sources at the expense of fresh groundwater within their territories (Goldstein R., 1996).

In the last 15 years, industrial development in Uzbekistan has increased sevenfold, and accordingly emissions of harmful substances have increased to 1.5 million tonnes, particularly from harmful chemical industries. Up to 1.4 million tonnes of mineral fertilisers and 80-85 thousand tonnes of various pesticides are used. Up to 1 billion tonnes of various wastes, often toxic, are accumulated in dumps and tailing dumps. The discharge of collector-drainage water, industrial, municipal, livestock and other poorly treated wastewater into rivers has reached 22-24 kilometres. This has sharply worsened the quality of river, groundwater, irrigation and drinking water. For some nosological units, in the zones of ecological risk, the population morbidity has increased 5-15 times, which requires urgent immediate measures (Razzakov R.M., 1996).

The Khorezm Vilayat is poor in fresh water resources. The main water source is the Amu Darya River and its irrigation canals-Levoberezhny, Tashsaka, Shavat, Polvan, Gazavat. The formation of surface and groundwater is directly dependent on the Amu Darya River. Any physical-chemical and sanitary-bacteriological changes in the Amudarya River water composition will affect the quality of water in water sources.

Observations of recent years show that the chemical composition of the river has changed sharply towards mineralisation, dry residue has increased up to 2.5 grams per litre, total hardness in some periods reached 18 mg/litre, chloride and sulphate content has doubled.

Water taken from surface water sources of centralised water supply systems in 55% did not meet the requirements of GOST on sanitary and chemical indicators. In some years, pesticide residues were detected in water samples from open water sources: 46.4 per cent in 1990, 40.3 per cent in 1991, 33.6 per cent in 1992, 34.1 per cent in 1993, 12.3 per cent in 1994, 32.5 per cent in 1995, 25.8 per cent in 1996, 48.6 per cent in 1997, 48.4 per cent in 1998 and 40.3 per cent in 1999. Open water sources still pose an epidemiological hazard, so in 1999 34.4% of water from open water sources deviated from GOST in sanitary and bacteriological indicators. Every year cholera-like vibrio (Cholera vibrio) is detected in 15 per cent of water samples from open water sources.

Ground fresh water reserves are very scarce in the vilayat. All reserves are concentrated in the canal and riverine channels and are mainly formed at the expense of surface water. The largest water source is the underground lenses of Chalysh fresh water deposit along the left bank of the Amudarya River, as well as small and medium reserves along the canal banks - Tashsaka, Shavat, Polvan, Kilichbai. Drilled artesian wells of Chalysh underground lens field in 1970-1980, were located 300-400 metres from the Amudarya river bank, but nowadays the river floodplain has moved away to a distance of 3 km from the artesian wells. Irrational use of territories of the second belt of the sanitary protection zone, absence of recharging water source, sanding of artesian wells, reduction of water flow rate led to the fact that water became highly mineralised, sometimes reaching up to 1.8 grams/litre of dry residue; total hardness from 9 to 15 mg/eq. litre.

Similar fate befell groundwater along Tashsaka, Shavat, Polvan canals. Groundwater reserves formed by atmospheric precipitation, which in Khorezm Vilayat are insignificant, and their flow rate is very low, besides water is not highly mineralised - dry residue in water reaches 3 grams/litre and total hardness up to 21 mmol/litre (Shavat canal). Such artesian wells in the vilayat are few and as a rule are used mainly for technical purposes, but in some settlements due to lack of other water sources, such water is used for household drinking purposes.

The physico-chemical composition of groundwater has changed dramatically, and its formation is influenced by precipitation, subsurface water composition and the physico-chemical composition of the soil itself. High mineralisation of subsoil water and soil salinity have resulted in groundwater mineralisation ranging from 1.5 to 50 grams/litre and total hardness reaching 30 mg/eq. litre.

Drinking water supply in Vilayat improved after the commissioning of the first start-up complex in 1990 and the second start-up complex the Tuyamuyun water supply system with a total capacity of 200 thousand cubic metres of tap water per day.

1992 of the Tuyamuyun water pipeline with a total capacity of 200 thousand cubic metres of tap water per day. Before 2000, there were 48 water pipelines in the vilayat,

of which 14 (58.3 per cent) did not meet sanitary and hygienic requirements. Due to lack of necessary complexes it was 186 thousand cubic metres per day, water consumption of the population in cities and district centres was 120 litres, in rural areas 50 litres. The coverage of the population of Vilayat with centralised tap water was 44.7%, including 60-70% in cities and district centres and 15-20% in rural areas.
Indicators of drinking water that do not meet the sanitary and chemical requirements of GOST were 58.4% and sanitary and bacteriological requirements 24.7%, hygienic indicator of water was characterised by a high content of dry residue, which in some periods of the year reached up to 2 grams per litre, total hardness ranged from 10 to 18 mg/eq per litre, as well as low-water periods of the year up to 20 mg/eq per litre. Sanitary violations in the operation of water supply facilities, low water availability and water consumption of the population, and high water salinity affected the health of the population. Thus, the general medical examination of the population of the vilayat conducted in 1988-1989 revealed that 72 per cent of the population in the vilayat had various health problems.
With the commissioning of the first and second stages of the Tuyamuyun water supply system, the capacity of water pipelines increased to 4,000 cubic metres per day; per capita water consumption per day in cities and district centres was 25% litres and in rural areas 80 litres. The coverage of the population with centralised tap water was 66.1 per cent, including 90 per cent in cities and district centres and 45.4 per cent in rural areas. The rate of non-compliance with sanitary and chemical requirements of GOST was 38.2%, and with sanitary and bacteriological requirements - 15.4%.
With the launch of the Tuyamuyun water pipeline, many obsolete water pipelines were dismantled and liquidated, modern water supply facilities were built, water quality and supply were improved.
The programme to improve water supply to the population of the vilayat continues with construction of the third start-up complex of the Tuyamuyun water pipeline, inter-group water pipelines in rural areas, etc. But unfortunately, there are problems here as well, the Tuyamuyun water pipeline does not provide for 31
Desalination plants, construction and installation works at the main water intake, laying of water supply network are carried out at a slow pace due to insufficient financing and lack of construction and laying materials, large diameter pipes, etc., which undoubtedly affects the sanitary-ecological situation. Unfortunately, the Khorezm Vilayat remains in the last place in the Republic in terms of water availability and per capita water consumption. The problem of water supply in rural areas is very complicated, as more than 34% of rural residents use well water for household drinking needs, these are tube and chess wells. As a rule, the depth of wells does not exceed 10 metres, mainly the formation of well water is due to precipitation and groundwater. High groundwater table and soil salinity determine the composition of water in wells, water in them is highly mineralised. Analysis of well water studies has shown that more than 69.2% of water samples do not meet sanitary and chemical requirements, where the content of dry residue exceeds 10 g/litre, total hardness up to

35 mg/eq/litre, nitrates, chlorides, sulphates exceed the established norm. Dangerous well water on microbiological indicators in water samples are found BOE-phages, which are indicators of subsurface pollution of groundwater. Excessive and irrational use of long-lived pesticides in agriculture caused migration of pesticides from soil to groundwater.

Changes in atmospheric air

The drying up of the Aral Sea leads to various negative changes in nature, including the atmospheric air. The annual decrease in sea level has resulted in the release of several thousand square kilometres of area. The open sea bottom over such a large area, has led to an increase in dust storms, especially in recent decades days with dust storms have doubled. They increase mainly in May-July, i.e. during the dry months of the year.

Human life takes place in the air environment surrounding him. The air environment ensures normal physiological processes of the organism. Air pollution can lead to pathological changes in the organism.

Observations from space showed that in one of the dust storms the area of dust clouds "stretched to 14 thousand square kilometres of land from such a cloud" fell 24 tonnes of dust. In another case, the area of the "dust cloud" was 45 thousand square kilometres. Dust storms spread over several thousand kilometres and lead to the deterioration of the ecological state of these places. Taking into account the fact that for decades tens of thousands of tonnes of chemicals, mineral fertilisers, pesticides and other harmful, hard-to-decompose chemical substances flowed to the sea with the waters of rivers and settled on the bottom of the sea, one can easily guess that there are a lot of harmful substances in the composition of dust storms. Every year 72 thousand tonnes of dust rise from the sea bottom, the total amount of salts is up to 170 million tonnes. The composition of salts is mainly chlorides and sulphates and they, settling on the lands of Priaralie and other adjacent territories, negatively affect the landscape of the area and lead to salinisation of fertile lands (Alibekov L. 1994).

In Khorezm Vilayat there are no sources of pollution of atmospheric air and external environment by toxic industrial wastes. There are more than 200 stationary sources of atmospheric air pollution on the territory of the vilayat, one of the major ones being cotton processing enterprises and construction industry enterprises. Basically, all cotton plants are located in the residential zone, organic and inorganic dust of which pollutes the appearance of settlements and causes environmental damage to residential buildings and public health. The annual emission of all enterprises together with motor transport amounts to one thousand tonnes. Samples taken from the atmospheric air of settlements show exceeding of maximum permissible concentrations of dust. Widespread use of pesticides in agriculture in previous years led to their migration in the environment, including the atmospheric air, they are detected in the air sample.

Changes in flora and fauna

Decrease of the Aral Sea level led to desertification and the Syr Darya delta vegetation decreased by 10 times and the Amu Darya delta by 251 thousand hectares, fertility decreased by 5 times. The change of vegetation cover was the most terrible, the place of perennial tukai plants was taken by one-year shura ephemera.

In the early 80s, the total area of saline lands in the Amu Darya and Syr Darya deltas increased 2-3 times compared to the 60s. Only in the lower reaches of Syrdarya in 1978, 114 thousand hectares of aluvial pasture lands became desertified and turned into saline lands. 732 thousand hectares of fertile land became unsuitable for agriculture.

Until 1960, the Amu Darya and Syr Darya delta had very many lakes, swamps and tukai. Reeds grew on large areas. Reed thickets in the Amudarya delta occupied 800000 and in the Syrdarya delta 250000 hectares of land. The most regional representatives of flora and fauna existed there. Besides, only in the delta of the Syrdarya River and the adjacent valley there were hayfields on more than 2 million hectares of land. Several hundred thousand cattle and small horned cattle were kept here annually. The flora of the Amu Darya delta was very rich; according to scientists, 576 species of higher plants grew there, 29 of which were typical for Central Asia.

The study of phytocenoses has shown that the state of this biosphere environment is also unfavourable. Residual concentrations of DDT and HCCH, exceeding permissible sanitary norms by 1.5-3 times, are detected in growing plant crops. In addition to pesticides, increased concentrations of iron, zinc, strontium, mercury, cobalt and other toxic elements are found in plants.

Since ancient times, the Aral Sea has been home to a large number of valuable fish species, such as moustache, carp, bream, pike-perch, the famous Aral roach and many others. An average of 450-500 thousand quintals of fish were caught annually from the sea. Under the influence of increased salinity of water, disruption of the connection between the sea and the lower reaches of rivers, i.e. destruction of the river delta, cessation of nutrient inputs together with river waters and other various factors, the number of fish stocks sharply decreased, as there were no ecological opportunities for their reproduction. Since 1980, from the sea for these reasons suspended fishing for the worse sharply complicated the life opportunities of the animal world, in addition led to the extinction of many species of them. For example, in Priaralie the farm for breeding muskrat has disappeared. If in 1950-1960 on average 250000 muskrat skins were prepared annually, in 1968 this figure was only 8000, and in 1978 only 72 pieces of muskrat skins were prepared (Alibekov L., 1993).

The dried up part of the Aral Sea makes up three million hectares of area, which has become the Aralkum Desert - made up of dust and salt. This mixture covers the entire territory of Central Asia, spreading through the upper atmosphere. Dust in Central Asia rises up to 9 kilometres upwards. At present, the vegetation cover is completely changed, there is absolutely no possibility of life for many species of animals, fish and birds.

PART 2

HUMAN HEALTH PROBLEMS IN THE REGION

Health status of the population of Priaralie

The aggravation of environmental problems of our time, in particular, the environmental crisis in the Aral Sea region, means the entry of mankind into a special period of historical development, which can be called the Era of Risk. Therefore, the relevance of theoretical development and practical activities to find ways to reduce the severity of environmental problems will increase.

In this connection, the special attention of the general public has been drawn for several years to one of the most acute problems of our time - the problem of the Aral Sea and the Aral Sea region, where the anthropogenic pressure on nature has approached not only a critical line, but has exceeded these limits. The tragedy of the Aral Sea is in fact a global ecological catastrophe. If the problem of saving the Aral Sea and Priaralie is not solved, it will be impossible to prevent the spread of the ecological disaster zone to new territories. The collisions in the interaction between society and nature that have arisen in the Aral Sea region affect the conditions of people's existence, social and economic processes of the present day, affect human health, and determine the main content of the ecological problem. The unheard-of grief did not suddenly fall on him, but slowly crept in, destroying people's health. More than 10 million people live on the lands directly affected by the ecological disaster. The level of morbidity of acute intestinal infections, typhoid, infectious hepatitis in the territories of the Aral Sea region is the highest and exceeds the national average by 11-14 times. The incidence of infectious diseases is particularly high among children under 14 years of age, including children in the first and second years of life. In 30 per cent of cases, these diseases are the cause of their death.

Changes in environmental factors, in particular, the chemical composition of drinking water, etc., have influenced the structure of general morbidity of the population: 70-90% of the population of the Aral Sea region (especially women) are sick with various diseases, such as cardiovascular diseases, gallstone and kidney diseases, gastric ulcers. The total mortality rate in this region has doubled in the last 20 years. Throughout Karakalpakstan, 80% of women of childbearing age suffer from anaemia. Over the last 10 years, the incidence of hypertension in this republic has increased 60 times and anaemia 550 times.

It should be noted that the relationship between the socio-economic development of the Aral Sea region and environmental disturbance is not direct, but mediated by the influence of social factors. The control over the environment in the process of development is carried out through certain factors. Therefore, the current environmental situation in the Aral Sea region makes us turn to the objective and subjective causes of the environmental crisis in this region. It should be taken into account that this crisis is the result of violation of dynamic equilibrium of the system "nature-society", extreme aggravation of its basic contradiction. The following processes are among the reasons for the violation of the balance between society and nature in the Aral Sea region: internal immanent activity of nature itself, which has a significant impact on people's livelihoods. This activity is intensified as a result of the development of internal contradictions of nature itself, which creates a danger of destruction for civilisation. In the case of the Aral Sea crisis, the increase of this danger as a result of human and society's own activity is new. Therefore, unpredictable immanent activity of nature acts as a response to the activity of society. Thus, studies by different authors have established numerous chains of interrelated phenomena occurring in different parts of the Aral Sea region and ultimately caused by anthropogenic activity. Let us mention the largest of them - for example, drying up of the Aral Sea and formation of a huge water body - the new Aral in the Sarykamysh basin, as well as such phenomena as waterlogging of lands, emergence of swamps caused by seepage of Amu Darya water from the Karakum canal, emergence of a dried strip and a centre of powerful dust outbursts and deposition of salt dust in the areas of oases and pastures. According to modern estimates, from 13 to 231 million tonnes of salts per year are accumulated on the dried areas of the Aral Sea bed. Because of this, the mineralisation of sediments in the Aral Sea region has increased by 6-7 times. Noticeable disturbances of ecological balance in the Aral Sea region and their negative impact on human health began to appear since 1970 and more significantly since 1973. One of the tangible signs of the impending catastrophe is the dynamic decrease of water flow in the Syr Darya, deterioration of its physicochemical composition and bacterial contamination.

It is well known that water can have both positive and negative effects on health. It is one of the specific factors of transmission of a number of infectious diseases. These conclusions are confirmed by the results of research on retrospective study of official statistics on morbidity for 1980-1990 (Kulmanov M.E., 1993). A comparative analysis of the dynamics of its indicators indicates that the Kzyl-Orda region of the Republic of Kazakhstan is one of the most unfavourable in the country for infectious diseases, especially intestinal infections. More than 4,000 cases of acute intestinal infections are registered annually, 76.8 per cent of them among children. The incidence of typhoid fever here is 3-4 times higher than the national average, and only in 1989 it decreased to 6.8 per 100,000 population (in 1980 - 45.1; 1987 - 37.4 and 1988 - 24.2). A high prevalence of AKI is characteristic of Ternozek, Karmakchi, Syrdarya, Jagalash districts and the city of Kzyl-Orda. Thus, in 1989, particularly high rates were registered in Ternozek district - 1150 6 per 100 thousand population (in 1985 - 1652.0), Karmakchi district - 960.4 (697.0), 38

In Zhanakorgan - 700.3 (537.6) and Kzyl-Orda - 906.4 (671.5) with the oblast 699.1 (866.1) and republican 411.3(573.2) respectively. Over the last 15 years, 36 major epidemic outbreaks of infectious diseases of aquatic origin have been recorded in the oblast. Thus, by the method of correlation analysis according to Pearson, a direct relationship between the deterioration of bacterial contamination of Syrdarya river water and the growth of intensity of incidence of typhoid fever ($r = 0.94$; $P<0.02$), viral hepatitis ($r = 0.57$; $P<0.05$) tuberculosis ($r = 0.76$; $P<0.005$) was established.

Statistically significant correlations of typhoid fever and AKI prevalence rates were obtained ($r = 0.88$; $P<0.005$), as well as inverse correlation of intensity of tuberculosis indicator with typhoid fever ($t = 0.7$; $P<0.01$) and ($1 = 0.66$; $P>0.5$) prevalence levels, and typhoid fever with viral hepatitis ($r = 0.66$; $P<0.03$) and tuberculosis ($r = 0.71$; $P<0.02$).

Compared to the average long-term indicator of infectious morbidity of the population of the Republic of Kazakhstan for 1978-1990, there are statistically reliable high levels of acute intestinal infections (including typhoid fever) and dermatomycosis. Statistically reliable high levels of acute intestinal infections (including typhoid fever), viral hepatitis, dermatomycosis and tuberculosis are registered among residents of Kzyl-Orda oblast.

Immunological studies conducted by the Research Institute of Epidemiology, Microbiology and Infectious Diseases of the Ministry of Health of the Republic of Kazakhstan and the Kzyl-Orda Regional Sanitary and Epidemiological Station revealed facts indicating a decrease in the level of immunoprotective system of the organism in people. Thus, in Aralsk the protective level of immunity against diphtheria, whooping cough and tetanus is not produced. In the oblast as a whole, the effectiveness of vaccination against tuberculosis has decreased to 75 per cent, and in some districts - to 85 per cent. There is a rapid progression of the tuberculosis process, which leads within 3-4 months to the decay of lung tissue. Consequences of anthropogenic impact on the hydrosphere of the Aral Sea region caused the expansion of the boundaries of natural focal infections on the territory of the region (plague) and changes in their landscape and biocenotic structure. There are cases of epizootics in the vicinity of 39
large settlements, including Aralsk, as well as cases of house mice involvement in the epizootic have been registered in residential floodplains of the Syr Darya.

The results of a number of scientific studies by some scientists have established that the chemical composition of water affects the development of some somatic diseases. According to WHO, about 80 per cent of diseases are related to factors of unsatisfactory water supply and unsanitary conditions of human environment. For the period 1970-1989, the total cumulative morbidity rate in Kzyl-Orda province increased more than 3 times, and ischaemic heart disease and bronchial asthma - 10 times, cholelithiasis and cholecystitis - 6 times. Increased morbidity shows that the intensity of indicators of many somatic diseases, widespread among the population of Kzyl-Orda province, is closely dependent on the value of the increase in the concentration of mineral substances contained in water. Thus, among the adult population the prevalence of gastric and duodenal ulcer, nephrosis, nephritis, IBS, hypertensive heart disease, rheumatism, glaucoma, cervicitis and endocervicitis had a high correlation with water mineralisation. The coefficient of determination ranged from 0.74-0.93 and $P<0.001$-0.05.

Among the child population (0-14 years old) a pronounced correlation was observed in iron deficiency anaemia, chronic nephritis, atopic dermatitis, congenital heart anomalies, rheumatism, infantile cerebral palsy, chronic rhinitis and nasopharyngitis with correlation coefficient fluctuations from 0.73 to 0.93 (P,0.001-0.005). The published in-depth analysis of long-term materials of Kzyl-Orda Regional Health Department of population morbidity for 1978-1990 allowed to establish statistically significant high levels of rheumatic heart diseases, cervicitis and endocervicitis, glaucoma, dermatomycosis, acute respiratory infections, typhoid fever, viral hepatitis, tuberculosis in comparison with the average republican indicators in the studied area. In addition, their intensity growth rates are significantly higher than the national average. Taking into account the fact that a significant part of the population of Aralsk and Kazaly districts lives in the epicentre or in close proximity to the ecological disaster zone, data on morbidity in Aralsk (base) and Zhanakorgan (control) districts were analysed. The latter is 600 kilometres from the sea, in the south-east of the region. It was found that among the adult population of Aralsk district there is statistically reliable excess of prevalence of contact dermatitis and other foroeczema, cervicitis and endocervicitis, tuberculosis, trichophytosis, schizophrenia and oesophageal cancer. The incidence of oesophageal cancer in 1988 was 14.4 times higher than the Union average.

It is scientifically proven that children's organism is particularly sensitive to the influence of a complex set of environmental factors. For example, among the child population of Aralsk district there are reliably high levels of iron deficiency anaemia and atopic dermatitis. In the Aralsk, Kazalinsk and Karmakchinsk districts, the incidence of hypotrophy and rickets in children is 6-8 times higher than the national average. Infant mortality has long been regarded as the most accurate barometer that reacts sensitively to the improvement or deterioration of living conditions. Thus, in rural areas of the region this indicator fluctuates within the range of 30.0-40.0 per 1000 live births, and its average regional level in 1989 was equal to 30.1. This is considerably higher than the national average (25.9 per 1000 live births in 1989). As a percentage of the total number of births, stillbirth rate increased from 0.7 to 1.0, and prematurity from 3.8 to 5.1, respectively.

Thus, the obtained data allow us to conclude that the critical environmental situation in the Aral Sea region, caused by anthropogenic impact on the hydrosphere, is the leading factor determining the nature of pathology of the population of this region, 41

Therefore, radical improvement of people's health requires cardinal solution of water supply problems, as well as restoration of ecological balance in the Syrdarya lower reaches and the Aral Sea area.

In Khorezm vilayat, medical assistance is provided by 152 outpatient polyclinics. There are 12 doctor's health centres, 163 feldsher-midwife stations, 120 rural doctor's outpatient clinics and 146 inpatient facilities with 7,610 beds. In addition, there are 8 sanatoria with 850 beds.

There are 13 State Sanitary and Epidemiological Surveillance Centres (SESC) in the vilayat (one regional and 12 city and district SESCs), which are equipped with modern diagnostic and monitoring equipment. The Khorezm oblast CDPHS has computer equipment, employs highly qualified specialists and has as its main task the sanitary and anti-epidemic control of the environment and the protection of public health. The laboratory service of the Central Sanitary and Epidemiological Centre conducts monthly monitoring of the external environment, analyses the movement of infectious and parasitic morbidity, and has a bank of information on the quality of drinking water, milk and dairy products and the dynamics of infectious morbidity.

Deterioration of the ecological situation in the Aral Sea region has led to a sharp increase in morbidity among the population of the vilayat. It should be taken into account that 47% of the population are children, 51% are women, and almost half of them are of reproductive age (15-49 years old) Therefore, the factors of ecological disaster affected first of all the condition of mothers and children.

In 1994, diseases of the blood and hematopoietic organs in children aged 14 per 10,000 population totalled 781.3 (313 in the country), an increase of almost 5 times over 1991. In 1994, morbidity among newborns increased twofold compared with 1985, congenital anomalies 1.4 times, 40 per cent of children were born with various deviations from the norm, and the stillbirth rate increased 1.6 times.

Maternal and infant mortality rates are still high (Table).

During the last years in our region among women of reproductive age there has been an increase in extragenital diseases (EGD), which in pregnancy adversely affect the health of the mother and foetus, the outcome of pregnancy and the future fate of the woman and the child. The combination of diseases of internal organs and pregnancy occurs in 60-70% of women. (Asadov D.A., 1992; Yuldashev K.Y. et al. 1997).

However, the development of extragenital pathology is associated not only with medical, but also with social and economic factors, standard of living, culture, society's attitude to this problem and other reasons. Often it is EGDs that are the cause of maternal and infant mortality, cause unfavourable outcome of pregnancy and development of formidable somatic complications.

EHS should be understood not only as diseases of internal organs, but also neurological, surgical, psychiatric, skin and venereological, infectious, oncological and others.

Taking into account the important place of extragenital pathology in the structure of maternal mortality, we analysed the prevalence of EGD among women of reproductive age living in the Southern Aral Sea region. Women of 15-49 years of age living in Urgench tuman of Khorezm vilayat were examined. Common clinical, instrumental (electrocardiographic, endoscopic, ultrasound, etc.), laboratory and socio-hygienic research methods were used (Abdullaev R.B. et al. 2000, Musaev M.R.et al. 2001).

At the beginning of the survey, 230 women of fertile age were registered in Urgench Tumen according to the lists of council villages and medical centres. We conducted a random representative sample of 20 per cent of the total number of women of fertile age, or 4393 women. Of these, it was possible to examine 3,311 women (74.4 per cent of the total sample).

There were 1,029 females aged 15-19 years (31.1 per cent of the total 43 examined): 20-29 years - 1186 (35.8%), 30-39 years -793 (24%), 40-49 years - 303 (9.1%). It should be noted that 1/3 of all those examined were girls and young women under 20 years of age. A large number of young women - is a characteristic of our region, where girls are married off early.

The distribution of women by social status showed that 804 (24.3 per cent) were servants and 716 (21.6 per cent) were workers. Housewives were 728 (22 per cent) of those surveyed, collective farmers - 334 (10.1 per cent), pupils - 596 (18 per cent), students - 11 (3.4 per cent), pensioners - 20 (0.6 per cent). Thus, 2/3 of women of fertile age are servants, labourers and housewives.

The normosthenic type of physique was found in 1421 (42.9%) women, asthenic - in 1260 (38%) of the examined, and hypersthenic - in 630 (19.1%).

Anaemia, gastrointestinal tract and kidney diseases are more common in the surveyed women of fertile age. In addition, the prevalence of oral diseases (caries, periodontitis, etc.) is high ($P<0.001$). More than half of the subjects had diseases of two or three systems. Table 8

It should be noted that high prevalence of diseases of gastrointestinal tract, kidneys is typical not only for women, but for the whole population living in ecologically unfavourable conditions of the Aral Sea region. Apparently, this is due to the poor quality of drinking water, its increased mineralisation (up to 4 times), increased chloride and sulphate content (up to 1.5-2 times) and hardness, as well as other factors related to drinking water (Iskandarova Sh.T., 1999).

Of 1,610 women with diseases of the digestive system, chronic gastritis was detected in 1,047 (65 per cent), chronic cholecystitis in 440 (27.3 per cent), chronic enterocolitis in 144 (9 per cent), peptic ulcer disease of the stomach and duodenum in 12-(7,87%), chronic hepatitis - in 103 6.3%), chronic pancreatitis - in 47 (2.9%), non-specific ulcerative colitis - in 18 (1.1%), liver cirrhosis - in 14 (0.3%) of the examined patients.

A combination of two or three diseases was found in 329 subjects, representing 20.4% of the total number of patients with digestive system diseases.

So, the majority of patients with diseases of the digestive system have chronic gastritis. The percentage of patients with chronic cholecystitis is high (27.3%). It should be emphasised that chronic diseases of digestive system prevail among all diseases. Pregnancy was detected in 445 (13.4) of the 3,311 women examined at the time of the survey. Thus, one of the main reasons for the high prevalence of EHS among women of fertile age living in Khorezm Vilayat is, apparently, economic and national peculiarities of the region, as well as unfavourable environmental conditions, deterioration of drinking water quality, non-compliance with the dietary regime and ration, violation of the immune system of the organism, frequent pregnancies and childbirths. Taking into account the negative impact of EHS on the organism of women of fertile age and pregnant women, as well as on the development of the foetus, it is necessary to recognise the health improvement of women living in the Aral Sea region as a priority task of modern medicine.

In connection with the environmental crisis, one of the major problems is the increasing pollution of the environment by potential mutagens, carcinogens, teratogens with genetic consequences. Thus, analyses of the incidence of congenital malformations for 1980-1993 increased from 5.9 per cent to 15 per cent among stillborns, and among live births it averaged 15 per cent. The range and frequency of congenital malformations were as follows: congenital heart defect 13.9 per cent, cleft lip and palate 4.2 per cent, Down syndrome 8.1 per cent, multiple malformations 6.9 per cent, hydroencephaly 12.7 per cent and clubfoot 14.7 per cent.

According to official data, the epidemiological situation in the vilayat is still complicated with regard to infectious, parasitic and contagious diseases. The incidence of acute respiratory infections remains at high levels, so that per 100,000 people the incidence of acute respiratory infections in 1992 was 710, and in 1993 and 1994 it was 606. The incidence of dysentery increased from 26.3 in 1992 to 33.7 in 1994. Children under 3 years of age are mainly affected by acute respiratory infections. The incidence of viral hepatitis remains at a high level.

The slight decrease in acute infection rates is explained by improved welfare, water supply, but in rural areas without piped water, the incidence of acute infections is very high.

There are 482 general education schools in Khorezm vilayat, of which 374 (77.6 per cent) are built according to the standard design and 108 (22.4 per cent) are located in non-standard, adapted buildings that do not meet sanitary and hygienic requirements. Water supply in 275 (57.1 per cent) schools is from piped water, and 207 (42.9 per cent) from wells, the water of which in 86 per cent of samples does not meet sanitary requirements.

Analysis of the morbidity of schoolchildren (age 7-17 years) shows that 20 per cent of examined children have respiratory diseases, 22 per cent have gastrointestinal diseases, 15 per cent have skin diseases and allergies, and 32 per cent have anaemia and diseases of the haematopoietic system. The incidence of genitourinary diseases in the examined children was 12.2 per cent. Due to insufficient iodine content in food products, 13.4 per cent of children suffer from endemic goitre; due to insufficient fluoride content in drinking water, 87 per cent of children suffer from dental caries.

There are 445 preschool institutions in the vilayat, of which 350 (78.6 per cent) are located in standard buildings, 95 (21.4 per cent) are located in non-standard, adapted buildings that do not meet sanitary and hygienic requirements, 262 (58.9 per cent) have piped water supply and 183 (41.1 per cent) have well water, which is highly mineralised.

An analysis of the morbidity rate of preschool children (1.5-7 years of age) shows that 17.7 per cent of the examined children have respiratory diseases, 16.8 per cent have gastrointestinal diseases, 10.2 per cent have skin and allergic diseases, and 28.4 per cent have blood and haematopoietic diseases. Due to insufficient iodine content in food and water, 10.2 per cent of children were found to have endemic goitre, and 74.5 per cent of children suffer from dental caries due to lack of fluoride or its insufficiency

in water.
To address the issue of preserving the younger generation, capital investments are needed first and foremost to improve the material and technical base of public education facilities and to provide children with the necessary environmentally friendly foodstuffs.
The unfavourable environmental situation has also affected the quality of nutrition of the population of Vilayat. The analysis of food products shows insufficient nutritional and energy value of rations, as well as the lack of ecologically clean agricultural food products. So the population of the region consumes meat and meat products by 22,7 % less than recommended by norms, milk and dairy products by 35 % less, potatoes by 45,7 %, consumption in proteins of animal origin meet their needs in food products by 60 %, urban and by 52 %. Very low provision of children with foodstuffs. So their needs in bread and bakery products are covered by 67,2 % of established norms on 17 % lower indicator of consumption of dairy products of meat and fish.
Insufficient consumption of micronutrients, especially iron and iodine, is noted in the diet of children and mothers. The unfavourable environmental situation has affected the hygienic indicators of foodstuffs, as analyses of 5.7 per cent of samples of meat and meat products, 5.2 per cent of samples of milk and dairy products, 6.6 per cent of samples of fish, and 5.4 per cent of samples of bread and bakery products revealed deviations from hygienic norms in 45.8 per cent of samples of foodstuffs.

Scientific research on public health and the development of interventions a new approach to diagnosis, treatment and prevention of "environmentally dependent" diseases.
of "ecologically dependent" diseases.

The constant deterioration of the environmental situation in the Southern Aral Sea region has led to the emergence of environmental, socio-economic and medical problems. Aral Sea region has led to the emergence of environmental, socio-economic and medical problems, the leading of which is the negative impact of environmentally unfavourable factors on the health of the population living in this region. Our ten-year study of this problem shows that there are practically no scientific works devoted to this direction. Exactly what unfavourable factors affect certain organs and systems of the human organism and the consequences of these phenomena were not disclosed. Besides, there was no information about the state of health of the sensitive part of the population - children and women of fertile age, about infectious diseases among children, about the course of diseases of internal organs among the population. Scientific research was required to study the system of organism resistance to infections and to determine it in a comparative aspect with the population of ecologically favourable regions of the republic.
It should be emphasised that expeditions organised by some foreign and central medical institutions research institutes are ineffective, as the studies are carried out without taking into account local climatic and geographical conditions, environmental conditions, do not cover the whole region, are short and expensive. In order to obtain

reliable, scientifically based results, it is necessary to conduct studies throughout the year throughout the region.
All these conditions are observed when conducting research by scientists of local medical institutions of the Republic of Karakalpakstan and Khorezm Viloyat.
In the Republic of Karakalpakstan, research work is being carried out in several broad areas, the leading of which are studies devoted to determining the immune status and health status of the population and studying the health status of girls and women of fertile age under the leadership of Professor Tursunbai Beijanovich Yeschanov, Academician of the Academy of Sciences of the Republic of Karakalpakstan.
In Khorezm Viloyat (Urgench branch of TMA) research works are carried out in several directions: prevalence, structure of the peculiarities of the course of gastric and duodenal ulcer disease among the population of different age categories and new approaches to its treatment; peculiarities of the immune system and intestinal microbiocenosis in healthy and diarrhoeal patients of children and new approaches to their correction; peculiarities of the state of specific and non-specific resistance factors to infections in pregnant women, maternity women and ways of their bio- and immunocorrection.
The results of these studies have been finalised and are being implemented in public health practice.
In studying various aspects of diarrhoeal diseases, we examined 539 children, including 179 with various diarrhoeal diseases of bacterial aetiology treated in 1994-1997. All patients were divided into groups: patients with dysentery -43 children, salmonellosis - 30, colitis - 34, diarrhoeal diseases of other bacterial etiology (DDDE) -23, diarrhoeal diseases of unspecified etiology (DDNE) - 49 children. The control group consisted of 32 practically healthy children of the same age. The control group consisted of 32 practically healthy children of the same age from Southern Priaralie (1 control group) and Tashkent (2 control group). The normative materials for Tashkent were obtained by Garib F.Y., 3alyalieva M.V. (1989). Then all sick children were divided into two groups: I- 107 children who received conventional antidiarrhoeal treatment, 72 children who were included in the complex of general antidiarrhoeal treatment with domestic preparations "Immunomodulin" (Research Institute of Vaccini Sera) and "Bifidumbacterin PL (MP "Orom" Tashkent).
In addition, 328 practically healthy and premorbid background children living in Southern Priaralie (Khorezm Viloyat) were examined before and after prophylactic bio- and immunocorrection, as well as long-term results (within 2-3 months).Among them 179 boys, 149 girls, 2/3 of the examined were from the city and 1/3 from rural areas.
On the basis of medical examination and anamnesis, the children were characterised as practically healthy. The examinations were carried out by specialists of the complex team (paediatrician, therapist, dentist, microbiologist). All children were divided into 6 groups: 1 group (58 children) received "Bifidumbacterin" produced in the Russian Federation as a biocorrector of dysbiotic processes of the large intestine, 2 (51

children) "Lactobacillus" produced in the Republic of Uzbekistan, 3 (55 children) - "Bifidumbacterin RG" of domestic production, 4 (57 children) - complex biocorrection with "Bifidumbacterin PL" and "Lactobacgerin" of domestic production, 5 (33 children with premorbid background) - complex bio- and immunocorrection with bacterial preparations and "Immunomodulin" in injectable and tablet forms, 6 (74 children) - bio- and immunocorrection (control).

The following dosages were chosen: "Bifidumbacterin", "Bφidym-baκτepinPL", "Lactobacillus" - 5 doses 3 times a day (for prophylaxis 2 times a day) 30 min. before meals for 14 days. "Immunomodulin" was administered intramuscularly 0.5 -1.0 ml once a day for 7 days, in tablets administered subligually 1 mg/kg for 7-14 days.

The immune status of children with diarrhoeal diseases of bacterial etiology was assessed by the main parts of the immune system: total number of lymphocytes: content of T-lymphocytes, T-helpers, T- cympeccopos, B-lymphocytes, FAN, FCH, immunoglobulins. classes A,M,C in 50

serum (Petrov R.V. et al., 1984). The results were compared with those of two control groups.

Bacteriological studies of faeces were carried out on the basis of the quantitative method and a special set of elective nutrient media taking into account the methodological recommendations of Epstein-Litvak, Gracheva N.M. et al. (1987) as modified by

Garib F.Y., Narbaeva I.E. et al. (1994). Faeces were collected in bakpechatki and delivered to the laboratory within two hours. Aerobic microorganisms were cultured on Endo Saburo medium, milk-salt agar and 5% blood agar, microasrophiles (lactobacilli) - on MPC - 4 medium in an exicator in a flashlight atmosphere, anaerobic microorganisms - on Blaurocca medium according to Nuraliev N.A. (1996). The isolated microorganisms were identified to genus or species on the basis of culture, morphological, tinctorial and biochemical properties in accordance with generally accepted methods and with the help of the "Brief Bacterial Identifier by Bergi" (1980). Bacterial counts were expressed in LgKOE/rp.

The studies have shown that in practically healthy children of the Southern Priaralie (1 control group) the content of lymphocytes in the blood is significantly lower ($P<0.001$) than in children of Tashkent city (2 control group). The relative and absolute content of T-lymphocytes is sharply reduced - 41±1.2% and 950±28/μl (Norsha-63±1.4% and 1819-40/μl). This is due to the deficiency of regulatory subpopulations - T-helper and T-suppressors. The deficiency of T-helpers was initially registered in practically healthy children of our region in comparison with children of Tashkent city-10,1+0,7 and 15,4+0,2% ($P<0,001$). In absolute terms, this difference was even greater 234±16 and 445±6/μL, respectively, i.e. 1.9 times lower. Similar indicators were found when analysing T-suppressors: their relative content in children of the Southern Aral Sea region was 1.5 times lower than in Tashkent children; the absolute values were 158±14 and 303±8/μL ($P<0.001$), respectively.

The total content of immunoglobulin-bearing B-lymphocytes in children from the

Southern Aral Sea region was significantly lower than in Tashkent children-20.4±1.3 and 24.6±1.3%, respectively (P<0.001); a more significant difference was found in absolute values: 473-30 and 710-34/μL, i.e. 1.5-fold lower. The total number of null lymphocytes in children of our region is 3.1 times higher than in children of Tashkent city (P<0.001). It is interesting to note that the content of Ig A and IgM in the groups (P>0.05), while Ig C was significantly lower in children of the 1st control group.
An important factor of resistance against infection is FAN. Children from the Southern Priaralie have significantly lower FAN compared to children from Tashkent-46.4±1.8 and 60.1±1.7 per cent, respectively, and the neutrophil-phagocyte uptake of microorganisms is also 2.4 times lower.
A statistically significant decrease was also found when the immunodeficiency index was determined - 1.34±0.05 and 1.90-0.05 units, respectively.
In our opinion, the state of the immune system in infectious diseases, including diarrhoeal diseases of various bacterial etiologies, should be assessed by antigen-specific cellular immune reactions. Determination of highly specific ASL showed that their number in practically healthy children of the Southern Aral Sea region exceeds that of Tashkent children (P<0.001). As antigen we used supernatants of cultures of Sh. flexneri (subspecies 2a). typhimurium, E. coli (serovar 0124). It is interesting to note that the number of ASL reacting with E. coli in healthy children of the Southern Priaralie was 2.1 times higher than in the control group (P<0.001)
Comparison of immune system indicators of children with premorbid background (different degrees of anaemia and hypotrophy) and healthy children from the Southern Priaralie showed even deeper secondary immunodeficiency: a reliable decrease in absolute values of T-lymphocytes, T-helpers, and T-suppressors.
Decreased FAN-32.6±1.4 and 46.4 1.8% (healthy children); decreased IID-1.06- 0.05 and 1.3±0.05 units (P<0.001). This is explained by more profound changes in the T-system of lymphocytes and FAN in children with premorbid background.
Thus, in healthy children of the Southern Priaralie there is a deep immunodeficiency characterised by a decrease in almost all indicators of the immune system. Apparently, the number of ASL reacting with bacterial antigens increases not only against the studied pathogens, but also against other pathogenic and conditionally pathogenic microorganisms. This in turn increases the risk of pathogenic colonisation of the gut. Deepening deficiency of the immune system in children with a premorbid background indicates an increased risk of infectious, including diarrhoeal diseases of bacterial aetiology.
The study of immune system indicators of children with diarrhoeal diseases of different etiology showed: the total number of lymphocytes in patients with dysentery decreased to 16.6+1.3% (1 control - 30.1+1.4%). Similar decrease of relative and absolute indices of lymphocytes in blood was noted in salmonellosis, colienteritis, DZDBE. It should be noted that the relative number of T-lymphocytes in diarrhoeal diseases of different bacterial etiology was significantly reduced to 29,3±1,5% (P<0,001), and immunodeficiency in comparison with 1 control group was found in

96% of patients; absolute content of T-lymphocytes
was 398±20/μL, which is 2.7 times lower than in the control group. The type of pathogen had a certain influence on the depth of T- immunodeficiency: in salmonellosis the total number of T- lymphocytes was 298 ±17, and in DZDBE 500+20/μl (P<0.001).

In the whole group of sick children, a decrease in T-helper cells to 6.9±0.5 % and 94±6/μl was noted (P<0.001). The most profound deficiency was observed in dysentery and salmonellosis (67±7 and 72±7/μL, respectively), the least - in DZDBU (134±5/μL).

The content of T-suppressors was similarly decreased: 4,3+0,6% and 5848 μl, which is 3 times lower than that of 1 control group (P<0,001). The greatest deficiency of T-suppressors was observed in dysenteritis and colitis (3±0.6 and 4.1±0.3%), the lowest in DZDBE patients - 5.2±0.7% (P<0.001). 53

Consequently, the detected T-immunodecytobesulovlenie decrease in the number of its subpopulations - T-helpers and T-suppressors.

In children with bacterial diarrhoeal diseases, B-immunodeficiency was more frequent in dysentery (179±22/μL) and salmonellosis (199±21/μL) compared with both control groups (P< 0.001). > The increase of "null" lymphocytes in children with diarrhoeal diseases of bacterial aetiology was significantly higher than in both control groups (P< 0.001).

It is interesting to note that IgM content was statistically unreliable in children, IgG content significantly decreased (P< 0.005), and IgA content increased (especially in patients with colitis and DZDBE - 1.4 times). This is obviously due to the increased need of the organism in the production of secretory IgA.

Children with diarrhoeal diseases had sharply reduced FAN and FCH scores, with a more profound decrease in colienteritis (3.90+2.2% and 2.5+0.5 units) and a less profound decrease in DZDBE (41+1.8% and 5.7-0.7 units).

The analysis of IID calculation shows that the most profound immunodeficiency is found in children with colienteritis, dysentery and DLDBE (0.91+0.006, 0.94-0.05 and 0.94+0.05 units, respectively), the least - in patients with salmonellosis and DLDBE(1.04+0.06 and 1.14+0.04 units).

In the blood of patients with bacterial dysentery, 15.4+1.1% of ASL carrying receptors to Sh-flexneri antigens were found. In patients with salmonellosis, colienteritis and DZDBE, the reaction with shigella antigens was low and was 4.2+0.8, 4.4-0.2 and 3.8+0.5% (P<0.001), respectively. In salmonellosis, a pronounced immune reaction was observed in 100% of cases with antigens derived from S. typhimurium, with an average ASL content of 12.8+0.7%.

In patients with coli enteritis, a pronounced reaction was observed with antigens. E/coli in all patients, which averaged 17.5+1.2 % (P<0.001). It is interesting to note that the content of ASL reacting with E.coli was very high (14.5+1.1%), i.e., probably the etiology of the disease in children was E.coli, was very high (14.5 + 1.1%), i.e., probably the etiology of the disease in children was E.coli, but (due to changes in the biological properties of these microorganisms under the influence of environmentally unfavourable factors) it was not possible to detect them by existing bacteriological methods.

Thus, in children with diarrhoeal diseases of various bacterial etiology, the functioning of the immunity system is deeply disturbed: the total number of T- and B-lymphocytes in the blood, immunoregulatory cells (T-helper and T-suppressors), FAN, FCH, IDD decreases; the content of null lymphocytes and ASL, specifically reacting with antigens of pathogens, sharply increases. Small changes in the content of immunoglobulins A, M, C in serum are explained by the short incubation period of the disease.

Microbiocenosis of the large intestine and conception in healthy with premorbid background children in age aspect. In healthy children under 3 years of age, the number of bifidobacteria was the highest - 7.0-0.6 Ig KOE/rp, (the lower limit of the norm), but slightly different from the age category of 3-7 years - 5.9-0.8 Ig KOE/grp, respectively. Lactobacilli counts were also at the lower limit of the norm in healthy children (under 3 years of age 3-7 years; - 5.85±0.9 and 6.2±0.6 Ig KOE/rp. In children with premorbid background the number of lactobacilli was reduced 10-15 times. The specific weight of bifido- and lactobacilli (25%) in healthy children of the Southern Priaralie was significantly lower than that of children from Tashkent - 45% (P<0.001).

Escherichia coli with normal enzymatic activity were isolated in 100% of cases in both groups. Depending on age, no significant differences were observed: 9.3±0.9 and 10.2±0.9 Ig KOE/rp in healthy children and 10±1 and 10.0±0.9 Ig KOE/rp in children with premorbid background.

The specific weight of lactose-negative Escherichia coli in the total microbial spectrum of bacteria was 9%, which was significantly higher than in children in Tashkent (7%). In children with premorbid background their number was similar in both age groups 8.9±1.1 and 9.3±0.8 Ig KOE/rp, respectively. Staphylococci were isolated with constant frequency in practically healthy (76%) and children with premorbid background (82%). Haemolytic strains of Staphylococcus aureus were isolated significantly more frequently in children with premorbid background, but their number did not exceed 10 Ig KOE/rp.

Streptococci were isolated in sufficiently large numbers. Cocci (sum of staphylococci and streptococci) in the total microbial landscape did not exceed the generally accepted norm. The number of bacteria of the genus Proteus in practically healthy children of both age groups exceeded the norm (5.6±1.6 and 6.29±1.3 Ig KOE/rp), and in children with premorbid background at the age of 3.7 years there was some increase up to 5.0-0.5 Ig KOE/rp. The content of fungi of the genus Candida in healthy children was 10-15 times higher than normal (P<0.001), in children with premorbid background it was higher by 2.3 orders of magnitude -6.9±0.8 and 6.7±0.9 Ig KOE/rp., respectively (P<0.001).

Thus, in practically healthy children of the Southern Priaralie, the quantitative and qualitative composition of intestinal microflora is disturbed: minimal threshold value of bifido- and lactobacilli, increased number of lactose-positive and lactose-negative Escherichia coli, microorganisms of the genus Proteus and fungi of the genus Candida. In children with an aggravated anamnesis (premorbid background) in 100% of cases, the number of bifido- and lactobacilli is reduced and the number of lactose-negative Escherichia coli is increased.

High segregation and growth of the number of Enterobacteriaceae and E.coli are associated with the deterioration of sanitary conditions in the Aral Sea area due to the environmental crisis, as well as the peculiarities of the Central Asian region: climatic-geographical, hyperendemicity for intestinal infections (Mamatkulov I.H., 1998), immunogenetic features of the local population.

The study of indigenic and facultative representatives of normal microflora of the large intestine in children with diarrhoeal diseases of different bacterial etiology showed a violation of their content.

Bifidobacteria. In all groups, the content was significantly decreased compared with control ($P<0.001$), especially in dysentery -3.9--0.3 Ig KOE/rp, colienteritis - 4.2±0.3 and DZNE - to 4.2-0.1 Ig KOE/rp.

Lactobacilli. Their content significantly decreased compared to control groups by 2-3 orders of magnitude ($P<0.001$). They were least in children with DZNU - up to 4.8±0.3 Ig KOE/rp, the most - in salmonellosis - 5.6±0.4 Ig KOE/rp.

Lactose-positive E.coli. They were reduced by 3-4 orders of magnitude, most of all in the DZNE group - to 6.8±0.4 Ig KOE/rp; a smaller reduction was noted in children with DZDBE - to 5.9±0.5 Ig KOE/rp.

Lactose-negative E. coli. The content was increased by 3-5 orders of magnitude in comparison with control groups ($P<0,001$). In dysentery and salmonellosis their number is the highest - 8.8±0.5 and 8.5±0.5 Ig KOE/rp, respectively, and in DZNE they are the lowest - up to 7.0±5.1 Ig KOE/rp. In all studied groups, lactose-negative Escherichia coli were isolated in 12.3% of patients.

Staphylococci. Their number changed insignificantly. No significant differences were observed in children with salmonellosis, colienteritis and DZNE compared to the first control group ($P<0.05$). Only dysentery and DZNE showed a statistically significant increase ($P<0.001$).

Streptococci. They were isolated in 69% of examined children. They were most common in dysentery and salmonellosis - 8.9±0.5 Ig CFU/g, respectively.

Fungi of the genus Candida. They were isolated in large amounts in dysentery and salmonellosis - 6.9±1.3 and 6.8±1.1 Ig KOE/rp, respectively.

Klebsiellae. This genus of microorganisms belonging to the family Enterobacteraecea was isolated from coproculture of sick children in high titres - in 72% of children. It is interesting to note that regardless of the etiology of the diseases, the number of Klebsiellae did not differ practically from each other in all groups ($P>0.05$).

Proteus. An increase in their number in the large intestine activates putrefaction processes and aggravates dysbiotic disorders. In all children these microorganisms significantly exceeded the norm, especially in dysentery and salmonellosis - by 3 - 4 orders of magnitude more than control groups - (P<0.001).

Thus, a decrease in the number of indigenic microorganisms and a statistically significant increase in the number of facultative representatives of colonic microflora in children with diarrhoeal diseases of various bacterial etiology have been established. It should be especially noted that in the Southern Priaralie during diarrhoeal diseases the dysbiotic processes of the intestine are aggravated, dysbiosis is characterised by a violation of the ratio of indigenic and facultative microorganisms.

To establish the role of immunodeficiency and dysbiosis in pathological processes in diarrhoeal diseases of various bacterial etiologies, we performed correlation analysis to determine the relationships between the main indicators of the immune system, as well as to study intergeneric and interspecific interrelated variants in indigenic and facultative microorganisms. The increase in interrelated variants between the indicators, the disappearance of "physiological" and the appearance of "pathological" relationships, which are not found in the control groups, indicates that in diarrhoeal diseases of different bacterial etiology, the immune system and normal microflora of the large intestine are involved in the pathological process, i.e. they participate in the process of sanogenesis.

We corrected the disorder of intestinal microbiocenosis with "Bifidumbacterin PL". The positive effect not only on the microflora, but also on the immune system was observed. To elucidate the mechanism of such action of bacterial preparations, we studied the immunoactive properties of the preparation "Bifidumbacterin PL" in the experiment on mice - at sublethal irradiation and acute toxic hepatitis. It was found that irradiated mice production of antibody forming cells (AOC) in 10.5 times 58 decreased compared with intact (P<0.001).

At intragastric administration of "Bifidumbacterin PL" the immune response increased 3.6 times in comparison with the control. In mice receiving disintegrate, the production of antibodylogenesis increased insignificantly - 1.2 times (P>0.05). "BiφidymbaκτepiPL" increased leucocyte levels by 2.8-fold compared to control. And disintegrate had no significant effect.

Thus, "Bifidumbacterium PL" corrects immunogenesis and leukopoiesis in irradiated mice when administered intragastrically. It was found that in mice with acute toxic hepatitis the production of AOC was reduced by 1.9 times and the number of spleen nucleus-containing cells was reduced by 2.2 times. With intragastric administration of "Bifidumbacterium RT" antibodyogenesis increased 1.8 times and reached the norm. The content of erythrocytes in the peripheral blood of hepatitis mice decreased 1.6 times, leucocytes - almost 2 times compared to the norm. After intragastric administration of "BiφidymbbaκτepiPL" the number of erythrocytes did not change, and leukocytes - normalised.

Thus, biocorrector "Bifidumbacterium PL" at intragastric administration corrects secondary immunodeficiency caused by irradiation and OTT, as well as stimulates leukopoiesis (Nuraliev H.A., Batirbekov A.A., 1999).

Given the peculiarities of the course and clinic of diarrhoeal diseases of bacterial etiology, their treatment is carried out in a special order and according to a specific scheme. The complex of generally accepted antidiarrhoeal treatment includes: general health regime, diet, etiotropic, pathogenetic, symptomatic, symptomatic, tonic methods of treatment. They are directed against pathogens and products of their vital activity, normalise metabolism and water, restore the activity of different systems of the body.

After the conventional antidiarrhoeal treatment (group 1), absolute indices of T-lymphocytes and T-helper cells increased significantly, but relative indices in children with dysentery, salmonellosis, DZDBE and DZNE did not change.

It is interesting to note that the content of T-suppressors did not differ significantly from the initial one in all groups of sick children (P<0.05). The concentration of immunoglobulins A, M, C in serum, FAN and FA remained practically unchanged (P>0.05). Single reliable changes in ASL indicate that the generally accepted antidiarrhoeal treatment practically does not affect the autoimmune process developing in diarrhoeal diseases of various bacterial etiology. Calculation of IID and BAT showed the absence of statistically significant differences in all groups of sick children (P>0.05).

In children with diarrhoeal diseases, 5 out of 25 determined indicators changed, i.e. reliable increase of indicators in the total group was 20%; in bacterial dysentery - 28, salmonellosis 12, colienteritis - 32, DZDBE-16, DZNE-36%. The study of intestinal endoecology also showed no significant changes in the number of indigenic and facultative microorganisms (P>0.05). A significant decrease of Enterobacteriaceae-Proteus and Klebsiellae representatives in all examined groups was revealed (P<0.05). This is explained by their special sensitivity to antibiotics and low resistance to various factors of exposure.

After application of "Immunomodulin" and "Bifidumbacterin PL" in the complex of generally accepted antidiarrhoeal treatment in children, relative and absolute indices of total lymphocytes, T-lymphocytes, T-helpers, T-suppressors, B-lymphocytes increased significantly (P<0,001), decreased - "zero" lymphocytes and ASL reacting with bacterial antigens from Sh. fl exneri. S.typhimurium E. Coli (P<0.001). It draws attention to the fact that absolute and relative indices of ASL to the pathogen that caused a certain disease are reliably reduced. Thus, in patients with bacterial dysentery, there was a decrease in AFL reacting with Sh.flexneri- to 3.4±0.9% and 63±17/μl (initial - 14.7±1.0% and 154±11/μl, P<0.001), but the content of AFL reacting with other bacterial antigens remained practically unchanged (P<0.05).

A similar pattern is found in salmonellosis and colitis (P<0.001). In children with DZNE, the relative and absolute values of ASL reacting with antigens from E.coli were significantly reduced (P<0.001), indicating that the causative agent of this disease is apparently this microorganism, although it was not bacterially confirmed. In DZDBE, the decrease in ASL was significant, although not significant.

We especially note the immunocorrective effect of "Immunomodulin" and

"Bifidumbacgerin PL" on FAN and OY, which significantly increased in all studied groups (P<0.001).
Significant increase of immune system indices were: in patients with diarrhoeal diseases of bacterial etiology, dysentery, salmonellosis, colienteritis, DZNE and DZDBEU 100, 88, 80, 72, 96 and 72%, respectively.
Comparison of the results showed that domestic preparations "Immunomodulin" and "Bifidumbacterin PL have a pronounced immunocorregulatory effect: they significantly increase almost all indices of the immune system (P<0.001)
The following changes occurred in the microbiocenosis of the large intestine after complex treatment with inclusion of "Bifidumbacterin PL" and "Immunomodulin": bifidobacteria and lactobacilli significantly increased by 3-4 orders of magnitude, and in groups with ssalmonellosis, colienteritis, and DZNE reached the lower limit of the norm - 9.1±0.3, 9.1±0.2 and 9.2±0.2 Ig KOE/rp, respectively. It is interesting to note that lactose-positive Escherichia coli indices did not change in the same way. The study of facultative opportunistic microorganisms showed that their number decreased reliably (except for staphylococci). Especially it is necessary to note the decrease of streptococci by 3-4 orders of magnitude(P<0,001). Klebsiellae and Proteus-5 orders (P<0,001); quantitative decrease of facultative opportunistic microorganisms concerned all examined groups (P<0,01).
The increase in indigenic and decrease in facultative microorganisms restores the balance between them in the large intestine and therefore normalises the intestinal microflora.
In our opinion, the origin of the strain also plays an important role in biocorrection with bacterial preparations, and the receptor apparatus of local strains of bifido- and lacto-bacteria is more adapted to local conditions. Taking into account the fact that disturbance of intestinal microbiocenosis in children occurs long before clinical manifestations and serves as a precursor of deviations in the clinical and physiological status of the child, depressed immunobiological forces of the organism and increased susceptibility to diarrhoeal diseases of various bacterial etiology, it is necessary to carry out preventive biocorrection ("artificial colonisation") with bacterial preparations taking into account the epidemiological situation. In the Aral Sea region, preventive biocorrection of children can be carried out without preliminary microbiological analysis of faeces for microbiocenosis.
During biocorrection we used biocorrectors of different production: 58 children were prescribed oral "Bifidumbacterin" produced in Russia, 51 - oral "Lactobacillus", 55 - oral administration of "Bifidumbacterin PL", 57 - complex biocorrection "Bifidumbacterin PL" and "Lactobacgerin", 33 children with premorbid background were given complex bio- and immunocorrection with "Bifidlumbacterin PL" and "Immunomodulin" in injections (17 children) and in tablets (16 children).
After bio- and immunocorrection, the indicators of the microbiocenosis of the large intestine normalised. Curation of children during the year showed that this was especially manifested in the groups receiving "Bifidumbacterin PL", and

"Immunomodulin". Taking into account the absence of significant differences in the indicators of the immune system and microbiocenosis of the large intestine in these groups, as well as the lack of bio- and immunocorrective effect in the group that received "Lactobacillus" we suggest preventive biocorrection ("artificial colonisation") to prevent disorders in the gastrointestinal tract in ecologically unfavourable conditions of the Aral Sea region to carry out a cheaper and more accessible preparation "Bifidumbacterin PL" of known strains of bifidobacteria.

The profound secondary immunodeficiency found in children with premorbid background serves as a basis for the inclusion of "Immunomodulin" in complex with "Bifidumbacterin PL". The use of these two indicators of T-lymphocytes and FAN.

The mechanism of biocorrection is the normalisation of the microflora of the large intestine and the negative effect on opportunistic microorganisms, in addition, the probiotic, affecting the lymphoid cells of the gastrointestinal tract, stimulates T-lymphocytes and FAN.

Thus, the direct, indirect and mixed influence of biocorrection on the activity of the immune system of the organism has been established. It draws attention to the fact that sublingual administration of tablet efficacy practically does not differ from injections, and by cheapness and convenience surpasses it, so for immunocorrection we offer this form of the drug. Prophylactic biocorrection reduced the incidence of diarrhoeal diseases by 6.3 times, total morbidity - by 3.1 times; prophylactic bio- and immunocorrection reduced the number of diarrhoeal diseases by 3.6 times, total morbidity - by 2.9 times among children with premorbid background.

As a result of the obtained data, we have formulated several conclusions: the immune system indicators in healthy children from the Southern Priaralie reliably differ from the values of healthy children from the ecologically favourable zone: decrease in the pool of T-lymphocytes, T-helpers, T-suppressors, B-lymphocytes, FAN, FCH, 120 in the blood serum; increase in "zero" lymphocytes and ASL, reacting with antigens from Sh. flexneri, S. typhimurium, E. coli. coli;

- immune system indicators in children with premorbid background in the same region are characterised by deeper immunodeficiency: sharp suppression of the T-lymphocyte system and FAN compared to healthy children.
- deep immunodeficiency in children with various diarrhoeal diseases of bacterial aetiology has been revealed. The depth of immunodeficiency depends on the etiology of the disease. The determination of ASL is sensitive
a method of immunodiagnosis of diarrhoeal diseases.
- In practically healthy, pre-morbid children, dysbiotic changes in the large intestine, disruption of the quantitative balance of indigenic (bifido- and lactobacilli, lactose-positive Escherichia coli) and facultative opportunistic pathogens were noted.
bacilli) and facultative opportunistic pathogens.
(lactose-negative Escherichia coli, staphylo- and streptococci, Candida, Klebsiellae, Proteus) microorganisms.
- in children with diarrhoeal diseases of bacterial aetiology, dysbiotic disorders of the

large intestine are aggravated and lead to a complicated course of the disease, as well as reinfection.
- conventional anti-diarrhoeal treatment did not have a bio- and immunocorregulatory effect. Positive shifts in the activity of the immune system and the state of microflora of the large intestine were not observed. - Inclusion of "Bifidumbacgerin PL" and "Immunomodulin" in the complex of general anti-diarrhoeal treatment normalised the indices of the immune system and microbiocenosis of the large intestine. The immunoactive property of "Bifidumbacterin PL" was established in the experiment on mice.
- prophylactic biocorrection ("artificial colonisation") "Bifidumbacgerin PL" in practically healthy children had a positive effect on the immune system and intestinal microbiocenosis indicators: it reduced the frequency of diarrhoeal diseases by 6.3 times.
- application of "Bifidumbacgerin PL" and the tablet form of "Immunomodulin" for prophylactic bio- and immunocorrection in children with premorbid background had immunostimulating and biocorrective effects: the frequency of diarrhoeal diseases in these children decreased by 3.6 times. From the above, the following recommendations for practical health care follow.
The introduction of "Immunomodulin" 0.5-1.0 ml once a day intramuscularly for 7 days and "Bifidumbacterin PL" 5 doses 3 times a day for 14 days 30 min before meals has a pronounced immunocorrective, biocorrective and clinical effect. To determine the immune status of children, an additional criterion-immunodeficiency index (IDI) is proposed, with the help of which the depth of immunodeficiency is clearly defined. Ero is used for laboratory diagnosis of diarrhoeal diseases. For the determination of bifidobacteria it is suggested to grow them under CO, burning candle atmosphere in an exicator for 48-72 hours on a dense nutrient medium. In order to prevent various diarrhoeal diseases of bacterial etiology among practically healthy children up to 7 years of age it is necessary to carry out preventive biocorrection ("artificial colonisation") with the preparation "Bifidumbacterin PL "no 5 doses 2 times a day for 14 days orally for 30 min. before meals; among children with premorbid background combined bio- and immunocorrection with "Bifidumbaктеpin PL" (same doses and terms) and "Immunomodulin" in tablets 1 mg/kg for 7-14 days (Nuraliev N.A., 2001).
The next direction of our scientific research was the study of morbidity, as well as the determination of intestinal microbiocenosis and immune system activity in first-born women (Matnazarova G.S., 1999).
Preliminary analysis of the causes of high morbidity among women of fertile age shows that anaemia in women of reproductive age is not related to the frequency of pregnancy and childbirth, but is a consequence of chronic foci of infection and pathology of internal organs, primarily the GI tract, kidneys and others.
The analysis of the conducted studies allows us to conclude that the most frequent among women of reproductive age living in the region (71.1%), as well as a significant proportion of diseases of the gastrointestinal tract, mainly inflammatory

genesis. Pathology of the gastrointestinal tract in 98% of cases is accompanied by the development of anaemia, which indicates the presence of nutritional factor in the genesis of the latter in women of reproductive age living in the zone of Southern Priaralie.

In this case, apparently, an important role is played by environmentally unfavourable factors associated with the ongoing drying up of the Aral Sea, especially the deterioration of the quality of drinking water, food and others, which affect not only the hematopoiesis system, the state of the gastrointestinal tract, but also the body as a whole, including the immune system.

Based on the above, we assumed the presence of a combined disorder of intestinal microbiocenosis and immune system in the genesis of anaemia in primiparous women, which justified our further studies.

The state of intestinal microflora was studied in 148 first-pregnant pregnant women, of whom 72 women were diagnosed with HDA P degree (Hb 90 to 71 g/l), 57 women with HDA W degree (Hb below 70 g/l), and 19 healthy (without HDA, Hb 111 and above) first-pregnant pregnant women constituted the control group. All women were examined on admission and at discharge from hospital, i.e. after treatment.

First-born pregnant women without anaemia (haemoglobin content more than 110 g/l) were examined in the dynamics of the gestational period: in the [trimester (16 to 27 weeks) - 6, in the II trimester (28 to 37 weeks) - 7 and 1-2 weeks before delivery (38-40 weeks) - 6.

It was found that in pregnant women of the control group the character of intestinal microbiocenosis with increasing gestational age practically does not change. We can only note a tendency to decrease the number of indigenic microorganisms. Thus, the content of bifidobacteria decreased from 9.98±0.96 Lg KOE/r to 9.49±0.74 Le KOE/r (P>0.05), lactobacilli from 10.48±0.61 Lg KOE/r to 10.18±0.94 Lg KOE/r (P>0.05). There was an increase in the number of Proteus bacteria from 3.42±0.54 to 4.20±0.42 (P<0.05), indicating the development of putrefactive processes in the large intestine in the last trimester of pregnancy.

Some increase in other representatives of facultative microflora is observed. Thus, the population of lactose-negative Escherichia coli increases from 4.48±0.43 Ig KOE/r to 5.27±0.43 Ig KOEL, and fungi of the genus Candida from 4.72±0.99 to 5.14±0.83 Ig KOE/r.

The content of aerobic forms of St. aureus was stable (FROM 4.71±0.84 to 4.76±0.88 Ig KOE/r, P>0.05), and the number of Streptococcuss increased, but not reaching the values of reliability (from 5.37±0.5 to 6.51±0.93 Ig KOE/t, P>0.05).

Thus, the studies of intestinal microbiocenosis in first-born women with physiological pregnancy allowed us to establish that the species composition of intestinal microflora in the dynamics of the gestational period has a stable character. However, quantitative analysis of changes in the intestinal microbiocenosis in the control group revealed the presence of dysbacteriosis of I and P degree in 57% of the examined, the frequency of which increases in the dynamics of pregnancy from 20% in 16-27 weeks to 100% in

38-40 weeks. The high frequency of dysbiotic disorders of the large intestine is probably associated with the negative impact on the organism of a number of environmental factors (water and food quality, soil and air pollution, etc.) that depress the immune system, hematopoietic systems, and the normal microflora of various biotopes of the organism, including the intestine.

Changes in the intestinal microflora depended on the severity of anaemia: upon admission to the hospital, all patients suffering from moderately severe GID were diagnosed with dysbacteriosis, which was characterized by a decrease in the indicators of normal microflora of the large intestine compared to indicators of healthy pregnant women without GID. Analysing the obtained 67

The results of the studies, we were interested to know the state of the large intestinal microflora in first-time mothers with WID by trimesters of the gestational period. All examined women were divided into 3 groups according to the gestational period | group - 16-27 weeks - 47 women (31.8%); I group - 28-37 weeks - 35 women (23.6%); PT group - 38-40 weeks. - 35 women (23.6%); PT group - 38-40 weeks. - 47 women (31.8%). The results indicate that the number of indigeneous microorganisms (bifido- and lactobacilli, lactose-positive Escherichia coli) gradually decreases depending on the gestational age.

We conducted a post-treatment examination of pregnant women suffering from WDD. For this purpose, all women were divided into 4 groups. Group I consisted of 58 pregnant women with moderate anaemia and Group II consisted of 39 pregnant women diagnosed with severe anaemia. Pregnant women

Group II received conventional anti-anaemic therapy, which included iron-containing preparations: ferroplex, ferrum-lek, vitamins B, C, A, folic acid, glucose 10% or 20% intravenously (Hb below 70 g/l) after 36-37 weeks - plasma and erythrocyte transfusion. Group III included 14 pregnant women with mild-to-moderate WD in GU - 18 pregnant women with severe anaemia, to whom the antianaemic therapy was supplemented with the administration of "Bifidumbacterin PL" and immunocorrector of domestic production - "Immunomodulin".

As a result of the studies it was found that the traditional treatment does not affect the intestinal microbiocenosis. In the dynamics of treatment practically does not change the quantitative composition of indigeneous flora, in both groups there is a tendency to increase the number of pathogenic staphylococci in group [group up to 6.83±0.97 Ig KOE/r (P<0.05), Bo II group - up to 7.02±0.43 Ig KOE/r (P<0.001), which is significantly different in relation to Kana4OTH4HOMy index of the control group, The increased number of haemolytic streptococci, bacteria of the genus Proteus and fungi remains 68

Candida genus (P<0.05). In severe WDD, despite the treatment, the number of lactose-negative E.coli increased significantly up to 6.98±0.8 Ig KOE/r with a norm of 5.07+0.54 (P<0.05). The number of bacteria of Proteus genus also increased (deepening of putrefactive processes in the large intestine, accumulation of gases, which in turn may prevent absorption and utilisation of exogenous iron, thus

aggravating anaemia).
Conducted microbiological studies of the flora of the large intestine in first-born pregnant women living in the zone of ecological disadvantage of the Southern Priaralie show that 57% of first-born women with physiological pregnancy have dysbacteriosis of I and II degree, aggravated in the third trimester of pregnancy and before delivery.
Pregnant women suffering from moderate and severe anaemia develop dysbacteriosis after 28 weeks of the gestational period in 100% of cases, and with increasing gestational age the depth of disturbances in the intestinal microbiocenosis increases, especially before delivery. These data indicate a high risk of infection in the mother and foetus.
Immunological indicators in the examined first-born women with physiologically progressing pregnancy, residents of Khorezm region, differ from those of the residents of Tashkent city and are characterised by a significant decrease in SD3+ and SD 4.5 cells, as well as inhibition of phagocytic activity of neutrophils.
The quantitative decrease of immune system cells also concerns the decrease of SDZ+ cells and its regulatory subpopulations SD4+ and SD8+ cells. In addition, in the same women there is a decrease in B-lymphocytes (3F3- cells) and phagocytic activity of neutrophils, which characterises the non-specific resistance of the organism. In first-pregnant women with WDD, deeper disturbances of the main links of the immune system were observed. In particular, the number of T-lymphocytes decreased 1.2 times (39.8±1.0%) compared to the control. The number of regulatory subpopulations (T-helpers and T-suppressors) was reduced. Their number was respectively 22.8±0.8 and 14.4±0.9% (in the group without WDD 26.8±1.3 and 18.8±1.0%)-$P<0.001$. The number of 3 F 3 cells decreased ($P<0.05$). Phagocytic activity of neutrophils was 1.3 times lower than in the group of primiparous women without WDA. With increasing gestational age, a deepening of immunodeficiency was detected in first-born women with WDD.
Thus, it has been established that in pregnant women suffering from moderate and severe anaemia antianemic therapy does not positively affect the dysbiotic processes of the large intestine, in connection with which the existing dysbacteriosis of II and III degrees persists to the time of delivery, which provokes complications in the course of pregnancy and childbirth, and negatively affects the health of the newborn.
Given the above, we concluded that it is necessary to supplement the traditional antianemic treatment with bio- and immunocorrective therapy in order to prevent the development of dysbacteriosis and secondary immunodeficiency. Inclusion of probiotic ("Bifidumbacterin PL") and immunocorrector ("Immunomodulin") in the complex therapy promotes normalisation of intestinal microbiocenosis.
Correlation analysis between the main parameters of intestinal microbiocenosis and the immune system in primiparous women with anaemia before and after traditional anti-anaemic treatment reveals an increase in the number of interrelated variants of intestinal microbiocenosis with the appearance of so-called "pathological"

correlations.
This indicates tension in the activity of indigeneous and facultative intestinal microflora. In addition, the weakening of "physiological" relationships after the traditional method of treatment is revealed, which indicates the insufficient effectiveness of the conducted treatment of intestinal dysbacteriosis. We note the fact that correlations are more pronounced when analysing intestinal microbiocenosis than immune status indicators. This indicates that the intestinal microbiocenosis 70
is more susceptible to pathological changes than the immune system in anaemic primiparous pregnant women living in the Southern Aral Sea region.
Intestinal dysbiosis of I and II degree is observed in 57% of first-born women with physiological pregnancy at 28-38 weeks. First-born women with moderate and severe WD of moderate and severe severity showed impaired intestinal microbiocenosis in 100% of cases with a high degree of reliability ($P < 0.001$). Dysbacteriosis was characterised by a reliable decrease in the frequency and number of representatives of the indigenic flora (bifidobacteria, lactobacilli, E.coli "lactose +") and an increase in the number of facultative opportunistic bacteria (E. coli "lactose", fungi of the genus Candida, St.aureus, Streptococcuss, Proteus). The following important conclusions for practical health care follow from the conducted scientific research:
the dysbiotic state of the intestine deepens with the progression of WDD and gestational age and is most pronounced with grade III anaemia in the antenatal period;
— in the genesis of anaemia of PI Sh degree of severity in first-pregnant pregnant women living in the Southern Aral Sea region is noted dysbacteriosis of the large intestine, and secondary immunodeficiency state;
— inclusion of bifidumbacterin RG. and immunocorrector immunomodulin in the complex of traditional anti-anaemic repannn bifidumbacterin is effective in the correction of intestinal dysbacteriosis and anaemia in first-pregnant pregnant women;
— a direct, close correlation between the severity of intestinal dysbacteriosis and the depth of secondary immunodeficiency in primiparous women with moderate and severe WDA was revealed (Matnazarova T.S., Musaev M.R., 1999).
The next important direction of our research was devoted to the peculiarities of clinical course, prevalence of gastric and duodenal ulcer disease in patients living in the Khorezm Viloyat belonging to the Southern Priaralie, as well as the development of new approaches to diagnosis, treatment and prevention of this disease (Abdullaev P.B., 2001).
It should be noted that gastric and duodenal ulcer disease (GUDD) is a problem that has been studied for many years (Vasilenko V.H., 1981; Kasymov I.Y. et al. 1996; Grigoriev P.Y. et al. 1997; Zakhidova M.3., 1999; Abramson D.J. et al 1991; Graham D.J., 2001). 2001). Ho, the lack of studies devoted to the degree of prevalence of the disease in different age groups, the influence of environmentally unfavourable factors on its course, the lack of effective methods of treatment keeps relevance of this problem.
To date, the ecologically unfavourable situation in the Aral Sea region and the

deterioration of health of the population living in this region under the influence of these negative factors are known according to the literature (Karimov I.A., 1997; Berdimuratova A., 1997; Kulmanov M.E. et al., Duschanov B.A., 2000). A. Berdimuratova A., 1997; Kulmanov M.E. et al., Duschanov B.A., 2000).

In this regard, taking into account the fact that the negative impact of environmentally unfavourable factors on human health is constantly growing, in the conditions of Uzbekistan it is necessary to revise medical views on many diseases, especially gastroenterological diseases, including IBD in the environmentally unfavourable conditions of the Aral Sea region.

Scientific works devoted to NBJD were carried out by many researchers, but they concerned mainly diagnostics and methods of treatment of this disease (Narbaeva I.E., 1994; Loginov A.S., 1997; Nazirov F.N., 1997; Stupin B.A., 2000; CheatumO.E., 1999). 1999). Some scientific works are devoted to the etiology, clinical manifestations, prophylaxis of NBJD (Elshtein N.V., 1996; Ratiyani L.A.). It should be noted that to study various changes in the organism at JDDD, experimental studies have been carried out (Karimov H.Y. et al., 1998; Daminov Sh.N., 1999).

But in spite of all conducted research works this problem is insufficiently studied, especially taking into account the ecologically unfavourable situation in the region of Southern Priaralie. The study of its degree of prevalence, structure, peculiarities of clinical course in different population, age groups of young men and women, men and women of mature age, elderly people, women of fertile age, as well as the issues of adapted treatment and prevention of CJDD, taking into account the influence of a complex of environmentally unfavourable factors on the pathogenesis of the disease, remain open. Thus, the analysis of IBDD in environmentally unfavourable conditions is an absolutely new problem, the solution of which is of great scientific and practical importance.

In order to solve the set goal, a total of 5211 patients and their case histories with peptic ulcer disease of the stomach and duodenum treated from 1989 to 2000 were examined. The study was carried out in three stages: at the first stage the prevalence, structure and degree of occurrence of peptic ulcer disease in different population groups in the population was studied using the nested-typological method. For this purpose, questionnaires were created, which included information about the course, symptoms of the disease, results of clinical, instrumental, laboratory investigations, number of recurrences, as well as treatment measures carried out. For this purpose, before the beginning of the study, the number of adults was determined on the basis of lists of makhalla, village councils and medical institutions, which totalled 24360 people. Then by means of random representative sampling we selected 20 per cent of this population, which amounted to 48872 people. Of these, we were able to examine 37387 people, i.e. 76.5 per cent. Out of this number of those examined, 2991 (8.0%) were diagnosed with NSCLC. In 1331 of them (44.5%) the disease was detected for the first time, and 1660 patients (55.5%) had suffered from this disease before.

At the second stage of the research we retrospectively studied and analysed the case

histories of patients treated in the regional clinical hospital 73
Hospital No. 1 of Khorezm Viloyat, which totalled 1,950 patients during the research period. These studies were conducted to determine the effectiveness of diagnosis and treatment, as well as to find out the turnover of patients to medical institutions. In addition, the time of hospital stay, the number of relapses per year and complications in patients were determined for comparison with the indicators of patients who were under our observation in the following years. There were more males (66%) than females (34%) among those examined. No significant differences in numbers were found between urban and rural residents. The patients were mostly young, able-bodied, 15-46 years old (83.8%).

At the third stage of research all patients (1780 patients) treated in the gastroenterological department of the regional clinical hospital No.1 of Khorezm Viloyat in 1993-1997 were under our observation. Out of all examined 70.8 per cent (1270 patients) were males and 29.2 per cent (520 patients) were females. The difference between urban and rural residents was small, 52.5 and 47.5%, respectively. WHO classification was used for age distribution. It was found that 33.4% of patients were males and young adults, 28.0% were in the first period (21-35 years), 30.8% were in the second period (36-60 years) of adulthood, 7.6% were elderly (61-74 years), and 0.06% of patients were elderly (75 years and older). The following results were obtained when the patients were divided into social groups: 36.0% (640 patients) were employees, 23.5% (418 patients) were workers, 13% (232 patients) were pensioners and invalids, 9.7% (164 patients) were pupils and students, 5.6% (99 patients) were housewives, and 4.3% (76 patients) were collective farmers or members of shirkatnye farms. In addition, 8.5% (151 patients) were conscripts.

All studied patients were diagnosed using modern clinical, laboratory and radiological methods. The final diagnosis was verified endoscopically. To study the clinical symptoms,
peculiarities of the course of the disease and to compare these indicators, the studied patients were divided into the following age (population) groups: 1 Young males and young adults, 2. Men and women of mature age, 3. Elderly and senile persons, 4. Women of fertile age.

In order to develop an optimal treatment regimen for NSCLC patients of all ages, they were divided into the following groups.

The first group of 1232 patients were treated with the generally accepted anti-ulcer treatment, of which 532 patients were treated with the proposed by us diet No. 1 Xz;

The second group of 72 patients who received the antibacterial drug bactrim in the complex of conventional treatment:

The third group of 84 patients, immunocorrector, tactivin and bactrim were included in the complex of conventional treatment;

The fourth group of 108 patients, immunocorrector immunomodulin and bactrim were included in the complex of conventional treatment;

Fifth group of 132 patients, immunomodulin, bactrim and local remedy -

magnetotherapy were included in the complex of conventional treatment; 7
The sixth group of 72 patients, immunomodulin was included in the complex of generally accepted treatment. The seventh group of 82 patients, to whom magnetotherapy was included in the complex of generally accepted treatment.
All clinical, laboratory and instrumental investigations were carried out before, during and after treatment; in addition, these patients were under our observation after discharge for a year (Table).
Generally accepted antiulcer treatment included bed rest, diet #1a, Bomeprazole, Almagel, Ranitidine, Metranidazole, in case of HP association Denol, Tetracycline Hydrochloride, in case of pain Nochepa, in addition Retabolil, Thymalinabromide, Meprobomad.
Modern methods used in medical practice were used for the study. The clinical method included the traditional scheme: identification of patients' complaints, subjective interview, palpatory and percussion examination methods. Diagnosis was made on the basis of classification proposed by WHO experts. Determination of the severity of the course of JDCC was carried out according to the proposed method with calculation of points (Abdullaev P.B., 2001). Endoscopic investigations were performed using an esophagogastroduodenoscope ("Olympus", Japan). Radiological studies were carried out with the help of X-ray apparatus "Sirescope" (Simens, Germany). Laboratory investigations were carried out using generally accepted methods. The secretory function of the stomach was determined using "Gastroscan" (Russia).
Traditional methods of nutrition therapy were used to study the diet and develop it. For this purpose, the main properties of local dishes, the technology of preparation of national dishes were taken into account, and national traditions of the local population were taken into account when organising meals.
The survey of women of fertile age shows that the course of the disease was mainly chronic (96%), acute course was 4%. It was also found that in more than 1/3 of women the duration of the disease was more than 5 years. If we take into account the fact that 92.8% of the examined women were aged 21-35 years, it is clear that the disease occurred at a younger and younger age. In 3/4 of the women, recurrences of the disease were one to two times a year. This difference from other population groups indicates that women of fertile age have a milder course of peptic ulcer disease. It was found that 25.7 per cent of women are under dispensary observation, and 18.3 per cent are not regularly treated, the reason being the low financial security of the family and the constant presence of an infant child in the family. The same reasons explain non-compliance with diets in 60.8 per cent of women, and 66.8 per cent of women do not undergo preventive treatment. The study of complications of peptic ulcer disease shows that stenosis was detected in 66% of women, other complications such as bleeding (26.8%), perforation (5.4%), malignisation (0.2%) were detected in significantly lower numbers ($P<0.002$).
Pain is an important clinical symptom of peptic ulcer disease in women of childbearing age. It is most often localised in the epigastric region (65.1 %), and in

smaller amounts around the navel and in the right iliac region (16.3 and 12.6 % respectively), 36.6 % of women associate pain with food intake as delayed pain, and 35.7 % with hunger pains. Half of the subjects complained of constant and the rest (40.9%) of dull pain. 50.1% of the women indicated that the pain irradiates to a specific location, 17.7% indicated irradiation to the back, 11.8% around the navel. A seasonal study showed that in 1/3 of the women studied (62.2%) the disease occurs in spring and 26.5% in autumn, and 54% of the women associated the pain with nervousness.

Analysis of the occurrence of dyspeptic syndrome shows that these symptoms were mainly observed after food consumption. Thus, vomiting was observed in 51.9%, nausea in 59.3%, heartburn. In 29.9% of the women. One of the important causes of vomiting was its association with pain (34.5 per cent). Nausea occurred on an empty stomach (25.1 per cent) and sometimes without reason (17.8 per cent). Heartburn occurred and was associated with pain in 28 per cent, unrelated to pain in 13.2 per cent, and during fasting in 12.2 per cent. It is interesting that some foreign scientists denied the role of clinical symptoms in the diagnosis of peptic ulcer disease, associating it with the absence of these symptoms in many patients, that is, they pointed to the latent course of this disease. But our results show that this opinion is erroneous for our region. If we take into account that vomiting, nausea, heartburn and belching do not occur in a smaller number of patients (3.3; 3.2; 3.2 and 1.9 per cent, respectively), the fact that in patients of women of fertile age dyspeptic symptoms occurred constantly. and clearly indicates its peculiarity. Our attention was attracted by the fact that only 1.6 per cent of the women's intestinal activity was normal, 30.9 per cent of the sick women suffered from constipation and 33 per cent from flatulence. Constant change of diarrhoea and constipation was noted in 1/4 of women. The fact that almost all women had a negative change in intestinal activity was noted. In our opinion it is not only connected with peptic ulcer disease but also with the negative influence on intestinal activity of ecologically unfavourable factor for our region - water factor.

Taking into account the great role of endoscopic and radiological methods of investigation in the diagnosis of peptic ulcer we carried out a comparative analysis of the obtained data. The results show that the ratio of gastric and duodenal ulcer localisation is 1:5,1, and the frequency of occurrence is 14,5 and 74,3% respectively, in the rest of the patients (11,2%) the ulcer was localised in both organs. When studying the location of the ulcer in the stomach, it was found: in the pyloric part in 29% of the examined women of reproductive age, in the small curvature in 723.4%, in the subcardiac part in 13.8%, on the anterior wall and in the antral part, respectively, 3% each; in other cases, the location was noted in the cardiac part, on the body, large curvature, and on the posterior wall of the stomach. In the duodenum, ulceration was localised most often on its bulb (55%) and posterior wall (20.8%). Interestingly, endoscopic examination revealed hyperaemia of the mucosa in 81.1% of female patients, while atrophy, erosion and hypertrophy were not observed in the majority of

women - 81.7; 82.8 and 61.4%, respectively (P<0.001). It is noteworthy that the majority of the examined women (84.3%) had healed and long non-healing wounds, but ulcers with large sizes (more than 1 cm) were found in slightly more than 1/10 women (12.2%), only 0.2% of the sick women had more than two ulcers. This indicates a relatively mild course of peptic ulcer disease in women of reproductive age than in other population groups living in environmentally unfavourable conditions.
An attempt was made to study these pathogenetic factors when studying the incidence of NCDD in young men and boys. The role of genetic factor was found to be low, the disease was most often found in a family with an average standard of living and wealth. Smoking tobacco "nasa" in 78
young men aged 17-21 years can lead to worsening of the course and complications of peptic ulcer disease. Other etiopathogenetic factors are eating outside the home, eating food of poor quality and violation of the rules of rational nutrition.
When studying clinical symptoms, it was found that pain in the epigastric region was more characteristic of girls aged 16-20 years (62.1%), no significant differences were observed in the studied age groups in terms of pain localisation. Acute pain was observed 1.4 and 1.7 times more often in boys 13-16 years old. Distinctive features of pain irradiation in the same young men were noted, so localisation of pain in one place (73.1%) was 14.5 and 22.8% more than in other age groups. Seasonality of the disease was more pronounced in girls (spring 62.1%, autumn 27.6%) than in young men (P<0.005). In terms of pain symptom characteristics, distinctive features were more frequent in young men 13-16 years old, which is associated with a young organism and early onset of the disease. No significant differences in this symptom were found between the sexes.
As in women of fertile age, the dyspeptic syndrome was more pronounced in boys and girls, especially in young people 13-16 years old. The detection of vomiting, heartburn, belching and appetite changes in 100% of cases is a peculiarity of our region, since according to other authors such occurrence was not noted.
Certain peculiarities were revealed at diagnostics by means of endoscopic and roentgenological investigations. In contrast to the literature data the ratio of duodenal ulcer to gastric ulcer was small, in boys 13-16 years old 1:2, in young men 17-21 years old 1:3,4, in girls 16-20 years old 1:3,5. Of the 2991 patients of all ages examined, NSCLC was detected in 226 males and young adults aged 13-21 years. Of this number, 45 (19.9%) had ulcer localised in the stomach and 171 (81.19%) in the duodenum. In comparative diagnosis between endoscopic and radiological methods, the discrepancy 79
was found in males 13-16 years old and females 16-21 years old. This was especially evident when determining the localisation of ulcer in the stomach and duodenum. It is interesting to note that inflammation of the gastric mucosa, i.e. hyperaemia, atrophy, erosion and amount of mucus in the stomach was more pronounced in young men 17-21 years old compared to other age groups (P<0.005). It is noteworthy that in patients of these age groups, the number of ulcers was the least. Thus, only one ulcer was

detected in 86% of young men 13-16 years old, 96.4% of young men 17-21 years old, and 92.9% of young women 16-20 years old. This is explained by young age, strong compensatory and adaptive mechanisms of the organism, as well as less exposure to various harmful factors.

When studying NSAIDs in elderly and senile patients, we took into account the presence of concomitant diseases, of which the changes in cerebral and peripheral blood vessels were noted by 19%, the disease of cardiovascular system in 17.5%, other gastroenterological diseases in 21.5%, diseases of genitourinary system in 21,7%, diseases of nervous system in 17,6% of examined patients, we also took into account the fact that 76,5% of elderly and senile patients did not smoke tobacco "us", 83,5% cigarettes, 78% did not use alcoholic beverages, so the negative influence of these bad habits at present for these patients was minimal. But 41% of elderly patients did not follow the order of rational diet, 37% followed the order of diet sometimes and 66.2% of elderly patients did not follow the diet. It is these factors that we identify as negative factors that aggravate the pathological process and contribute to constant disease relapses. The fact that in 67.5% of patients the duration of disease is more than 5 years indicates the long-standing nature of the disease. In elderly and senile people the pains were more often located in epigastric and right iliac regions, most often the pains were manifested after meals in the form of delayed and hunger pains. In these patients, seasonality was more pronounced (93.5%) than in other population groups (P<0.005). Attracted 80

Our attention is drawn to the fact that all male and female patients of elderly and senile age showed very weak or no clinical symptoms, so Mendel's symptom was positive in 29% of patients. As in other population groups this indicator was 2.5-2.8 times higher. The same pattern was found in the study of dyspeptic symptoms, i.e. these symptoms were weakly and rarely expressed, mostly they occurred after eating. The results of endoscopic and radiological studies practically did not differ from the indicators of other studied population groups, it should be emphasised that multiple and large size "giant" ulcers of the stomach and duodenum were practically absent among elderly and senile patients.

When studying the peculiarities of the course of JDCC in different population groups, it became necessary to study the incidence, peculiarities of the course and diagnostic measures in a comparative aspect, as it would allow to develop an acceptable scheme of diagnostics and treatment of the disease.

Pain syndrome has been studied in young boys and girls 13-16 years old, young adults 17- 21 years old, mature age men and women 21-60 years old, and elderly and senile individuals from 60-90 years old.

There were no significant differences in the localisation of pain in the age aspect. In all patients, pain was most often found in the epigastric region, which occurred in 53.9-62.7% of the examined patients. It should be noted that the localisation of pains around the navel was significantly more important in women than in men - P < 0,002 (respectively in women 21-35 years old 22,9%; in women 36-55 years old 24,2%; 56-

74 years old 25,3%). There were no significant differences between age groups in the association of pain with food intake. Acute pains more often bothered younger patients, and elderly and senile patients were mostly bothered by dull pains. Apparently, this fact is connected with changes in the organism of elderly people and the "old age" of ulcers origin. In terms of pain irradiation, no practically noticeable changes were observed in different population groups (P>0.05). Differences were not observed by sex. To, that in young men of 13-16 years old the irradiation of pain to certain places was 15-16% more than in other age groups (respectively 73.1 and 57-58%) is explained by more pronounced course of inflammatory process, as well as the beginning of ulcer disease.

Seasonality of pain in all patients is associated with spring and autumn seasons, which made up from 84% to 93% of the examined patients. It should be noted that the younger the organism, the less pronounced the seasonality, which is associated with the state of the organism, determined by the lifestyle of adults.

The Mendel's symptom is particularly revealing. It has been found that the younger the organism, the more likely this symptom is detected. Thus, if in boys of 13-16 years old the Mendel's symptom was positive in 80% of cases, in young people of 17-21 years old this indicator was 64,9%, and in elderly men and women the positive Mendel's symptom was revealed reliably less respectively 29,0 and 26,5% (P<0,001). In our opinion, it is inappropriate to use this symptom as a determinant in elderly and senile individuals.

Taking into account the successes of modern dietetics, we believe that the organisation of rational nutrition and diet therapy is an important factor for the treatment of the disease and reduction of the incidence of IBDD. While studying this question we came to the conclusion that it is necessary to make additions to the existing diet, taking into account local conditions. We improved and streamlined the conditions and rules of the anti-ulcer diet, then defined a list of meals for this purpose. The conditions and rules include providing the physiological needs of the organism with the necessary nutreints; studying the influence of nutrition on metabolism, activity of the gastrointestinal tract taking into account climatic and geographical peculiarities and national traditions; organising the anti-ulcer diet taking into account the nutrition of the local population;

ensuring the best assimilation of cooking technology responsible for these people in the preparation of dishes for anti-ulcer diet; providing the composition of dishes with a full range of nutrient composition and energy value; take into account the mechanical, chemical and thermal sparing of the gastric mucosa in the selection of dishes for anti-ulcer diet.

When developing an anti-ulcer diet, we used diet No. 1 Uzb together with diet No. 1a, 16,1. On this basis, we developed and proposed for practical implementation diet No. 1 Khz (Khorezm). This diet is used as an anti-ulcer diet and is recommended 12-15 days after the appointment of diets №1a and №16. The purpose of using the diet No. 1 Khz is mechanical, chemical and thermal sparing of the gastric mucosa and faster recovery of the organism with a sharp decrease in the recurrence of the disease. The diet consists of basic nutrients (proteins, fats, carbohydrates, etc.). In physiological quantity peculiarity are restrictions of table salt up to 8-10 grams, sugar up to 30 g. dishes containing rough fibre and inclusion of local dishes, which is habitual for these patients.

Energy value 2950 kcal. Nutrient composition: proteins 100 gr fats 89 gr (of which 1/3 vegetable oil), carbohydrates 293.7 gr net weight of liquid 1.5 litres. The weight of one day's food is about 3kg (table). The order of meals is fractional - 4-5 times a day, in hot weather most of the calories are transferred to the cool time of the day (morning and evening).

In addition, on the basis of diet No. 1 Khz we have developed a weekly menu, taking into account the place of residence of patients, the degree of food availability in the local population, the technological capabilities of food preparation facilities, and the financial status of the medical institution. Menus are prepared separately for medical institutions of the city and rural areas. It is recommended to include more Uzbek national and Khorezm local dishes in the menu for rural and district hospitals, which has 83

clinical and cost-effectiveness.

Taking into account the widespread use of "us" tobacco among the population of Central Asian countries, we were interested to know the influence of this harmful habit on the course of morbidity. There were 113 patients with peptic ulcer disease under observation, 50 of them used and 40 did not use "us" tobacco. 23 patients who stopped smoking "us" after admission to the hospital constituted a separate group. The results show (Table) a significant decrease by 6.3 days ($P<0.001$) in the length of hospital stay in non-smoking "us" patients. The same reliable indicators were obtained when studying the term of ulcer healing and the terms of disappearance of subjective manifestations ($P<0.05$). This indicates a negative effect of smoking tobacco "us" on the course of peptic ulcer disease.

The determination of the severity of the course of the disease is important for the successful treatment of patients with CJDD.

Therefore, taking into account the complaints of patients, clinical manifestations of the disease and the occurrence of NAD in different population groups, a special diagnostic card "Algorithm for assessing the severity of the course of NAD" was developed, which allows assessing the severity by points. The diagnostic card consists of two parts: passport and evaluation. The passport part contains the patient's data, in the evaluation part on the basis of the patient's complaints and clinical symptoms, the physician puts points by the examined doctor, then the points are added up, compared with the norm and evaluated (Abdullaev P.B., 2001).

This method makes it possible to assess the severity of the course of CJDD more clearly, which in turn improves the diagnosis of the disease and helps to choose the correct treatment tactics for the patient. The importance of this method increases in rural medical centres and peripheral medical institutions, where expensive equipment

and instrumental investigations are not available.
Together with dietary therapy, we carried out drug treatment of patients with JDCC. The patients were divided into 7 groups. Clinical and endoscopic 84
examination, HP determination, determination of gastric acid-forming function and immune system activity were performed before and after treatment.
The analysis of the obtained results shows that different methods of treatment have different effects on clinical and endoscopic parameters. Inclusion of bactrim, immunomodulin and magnetotherapy in the complex of conventional treatment had the most positive effect, so the terms of hospital stay of patients made 15,6±2 days, against 34,4±3,1 days in the group of patients who received only conventional treatment ($P<0,001$). The same indicators were obtained when determining the terms of disappearance of subjective symptoms in patients (respectively 2,7±0,3 and 10,6+1,1 days). It is interesting to note that in all groups there is a reliable decrease of the terms of hospital stay in patients than in patients of the control group.
It was found that in the fifth group of patients, where bactrim, immunomodulin and magnetotherapy were included in the complex, the best reliable results were obtained, indicating the choice of the optimal treatment scheme. It is interesting that the introduction of immunocorrector in the complex of treatment of patients leads to faster positive results than patients of other groups. It should be emphasised that the sooner the subjective symptoms of patients disappear, the sooner calmness and faith in recovery return to them, this leads to the quicker normalisation of other indicators. Reducing the period of stay of patients in hospital is of economic benefit not only to the state, but also to the patient himself in our conditions. We would like to emphasise that the terms of ulcer healing are also sharply reduced, in the fifth group this index decreases 2-3 times, in the fourth group - 2 times, in the third and sixth groups - 1,8 times in relation to the control group ($P<0,001$).In addition, the degree of relapses after treatment is significantly reduced.
One of the important factors is to increase the degree of HP eradication. It was found that the inclusion of antibacterial drug in the treatment complex accelerates and makes effective HP eradication. And the combined use of OL, bactrim, immunomodulin and magnetotherapy bring eradication to the maximum level.
When determining the basal and stimulated gastric secretion, it was found that total and free acidity after treatment significantly decreased to normal values, but it should be noted that in all groups these decreases were observed without significant differences from each other, indicating that there was no significant effect on the acid-forming function of the stomach of the drugs used in various combinations.
Determination of the immune status in patients with peptic ulcer shows that they have a deep secondary immunodeficiency, mainly characterised by a decrease in T-lymphocytes and phagocytic activity of neutrophils, although the relative number of B-lymphocytes did not significantly decrease, the deficit was observed in absolute indices, which indicates the severity of B-immunodeficiency. After anti-ulcer therapeutic measures many indices significantly increased, but did not reach normal

values, apparently it is connected with a short period of immunological observation. More pronounced immunocorregulatory efficiency was established in the groups of patients, where the complex of OL included immunomodulin and bactrim, as well as immunomodulin, bactrim and magnetotherapy, where the percentage of reliable increase in immunological parameters was 100%: The following conclusions follow from the above-mentioned:

— the peculiarities of the course of pain and dyspeptic syndromes, as well as the indicators of endoscopic investigations of NSAIDs in young men (13-16 years) and young women (16-21 years), in contrast to patients of mature, elderly and old age and women of fertile age were revealed;

— less pronounced manifestation of pain, dyspeptic and other clinical symptoms of JDCC in elderly and elderly patients than in other surveyed population groups of the Southern Aral Sea region was established, in particular, by lower detection of Mendel's positive symptom;

— to the etiological risk factors for the occurrence of NFJD in the region of Southern Priaralie, along with the violation of diet, smoking tobacco "us", violation of the ratio of aggressively protective factors, also include environmentally unfavourable water and soil factors;

— The diagnostic card developed to assess the severity of the course of CJDD expands the diagnostic capabilities of the disease and reliably reduces subjective clinical errors of the doctor;

— deep secondary immunodeficiency characterised by a decrease in T-lymphocytes and phagocytic activity of neutrophils was revealed in the activity of the immune system of patients with CJDD. The use of immunomodulin and tactivin had the same clinical and immunocorregulatory efficacy;

— recommended as anti-ulcer diet No.1 Khz, including Uzbek national and Khorezm local dishes, had a positive effect in the treatment of IBD patients in our region and significantly increased the remission period of the disease;

— on the basis of anti-ulcer diet No.1 Khz developed and recommended in practical healthcare menu - layout for 7 days separately for urban and rural medical institutions, taking into account the degree of food availability of the local population, technological capabilities of places for food preparation, financial status of the medical institution;

— inclusion of antibacterial drug - bactrim, immunocorrector - immunomodulin and local remedy - magnetotherapy in the complex of conventional anti-ulcer treatment of patients had a reliable positive clinical efficacy.

The results of the study conducted in the regional multidisciplinary medical centre of Khorezm region, Khorezm branch of the Republican Scientific Centre for Emergency Medical Care, Central Polyclinic of Urgench and medical associations of Khanka and Khiva districts. The case histories of 1000 patients with diseases of the hepatobiliary system in the archives of clinics in the Khorezm region from 2006 to 2016 were analysed. From them, the case histories of 239 patients with liver cirrhosis were

selected for further study and analysed thoroughly.
ABC-analysis is a retrospective analysis, the essence of which is to assess the rational use of money for a certain period of time by three groups. When medicines are allocated to groups A, B, C, group A accounts for 80% of total expenditure, group B for 15% and group C for 5%.
VEN analysis is used to assess the quality of evidence for the use of pharmacotherapy. The essence of VEN-analysis is the distribution of medicines used in a health care facility over a selected period of time according to the level of vital importance. This allows a formal assessment of the correctness of prescribing drugs for a particular pathology.
In a scientific study entitled "Peculiarities of the prevalence of diseases of the hepatobiliary system in the Khorezm region" conducted by researchers of the Urgench branch of TMA, the necessary information from the case histories of 1000 patients with diseases of the hepatobiliary system for the period from 2006 to 2016 in certain hospitals of the Khorezm region was studied retrospectively using pharmacoepidemiological methods. Of the total number of patients examined, 64% were women and 36% were men. The data show that the incidence of hepatobiliary system diseases in women is 1.8 times higher than in men.
In the course of the study, when analysing data on the place of residence of the patients, it was revealed that 62% of those examined lived in rural areas and 38% in urban areas. This indicates that the disease of the hepatobiliary system is 1.6 times higher among the rural population than among the population living in the city.
Analysis of the age of the examined patients showed that the average age of all examined patients in the region was 49.5±10.3 years. Considering these patients by age categories revealed: 1) minors, i.e. children - 5 people; 2) aged from 18 to 60 years, i.e. middle-aged - 835 people; 3) older than 60 years, i.e. elderly - 160 people.
In the study, the duration of treatment in the region was up to 10 days in 599 patients, 10 to 20 days in 363 patients, 20 patients 20 to 30 days and 18 patients more than 1 month. The data show that the vast majority of patients, or 96.2 per cent, were treated for up to 20 days. Only 3.6 per cent of patients were treated for more than 20 days.
The analysis performed by nosological types of diseases detected in these patients showed that out of 1000 examined patients in the region 142 were diagnosed with cholecystitis, 415 with hepatitis, 3 with hepatocellular carcinoma, 201 with chronic hepatitis and 239 with liver cirrhosis (Table).

Morbidity rates by nosological types in the studied 1000 patients

№	Name	Hole cystitis	Hepatitis	Malignant- tumour tumour livers	Transition of chronic hepatitis to CKD	CP
1	Khiva district medical association	56	80	-	64	49
2	Khankinsky Raion medical association	59	65	-	82	46
3	Medical institutions of	27	270	3	55	144

	Urgench city					
	Total:	142	415	3	201	239

Thus, it was found that the incidence of hepatobiliary diseases in Khorezm Province is 1.8 times higher among women than among men. In comparison with literature data, in the total number of patients treated for hepatobiliary diseases in Bukhara province, the proportion of women was 51 per cent, and in Navoi province the proportion of men was 55 per cent. It follows that there is no specific pattern in the frequency of hepatobiliary diseases.

Based on the above, it follows that during the study, out of 1000 patients with hepatobiliary disease, the case histories of 239 patients with liver cirrhosis were singled out for further in-depth analysis and analysed in detail at later stages of the study. Of the 239 patients with cirrhosis at the time of the study, 123 were female and 116 were male. In terms of age: 56 (23%) were aged 18-40 years, 138 (59%) were aged 41-60 years, and 45 (18%) were aged 61 years or older. Of these patients, 3.3% had higher education, 41.0% had specialised secondary education and 55.7% had secondary education. Of these patients, 33 % were urban dwellers and 67 % were rural dwellers. The results of the analysis of the duration of the course of the disease in these patients were as follows: in 28% of patients - from 1 to 5 years, 38% of patients - from 5 to 10 years and34% of patients more than 10 years.

A total of 1532 drugs were used during the study period. This indicates that each of 239 patients with liver cirrhosis took an average of 6.4 drugs. At the same time, when analysing the number (frequency) of use of all drugs by pharmacological groups, it was found that the highest indicator belongs to hepatoprotectors (Table).

Number of uses of all groups of drugs used by
Patients with cirrhosis

№	**Groups of drugs used**	**Unit of measurement**
1	Hepatoprotectors	534
2	Vitamin preparations	194
3	Agents affecting water and salt metabolism	155
4	Diuretics and saluretics	152
5	Blood and blood substitutes	103
6	Drugs affecting the cardiovascular system	95
7	Antispasmodics and analgesics	56
8	Antibacterial agents	39
9	Agents that improve blood circulation in the brain	37
10	Drugs affecting the blood coagulation system	32
11	Enzyme preparations	31
12	Hormonal drugs	24
13	Immunomodulators	22
14	Hypotensive agents	17
15	Other drugs	41

Total:	**1532**

This figure was 34.9% of the total number of drugs used and showed that each patient received an average of 2.2 hepatoprotectors. However, 15 patients did not use any hepatoprotectant and the used ones were used in 224 patients, it was found that an average of 2.4 hepatoprotectants were used per patient. This implies that the use of baseline drugs in patients with cirrhosis, was 37.5% and the remaining 62.5% were used as secondary drugs. This once again proves that due to insufficient use of hepatotropic agents it is impossible to achieve good efficacy in the treatment of liver cirrhosis.

It was found that 12.7% of the drugs used were vitamins, which were the second most frequently used, 10.1% were drugs affecting water and salt metabolism, and 10.0% were diuretics and saluretics. The frequency of use of other groups listed in the table was less than 10.0%.

Considering that the most commonly used drugs are hepatoprotectors and are the main study material in this study, the following pattern was observed when analysed by type of drug and frequency of use of each drug .

Frequency of use of hepatoprotective agents used by by patients with cirrhosis

№№	Hepatoprotectors	Frequency
1	Essential phospholipids	161
2	Riboxin	128
3	UDCC	59
4	Thiotriosalin	54
5	Carsyl	38
6	Apkasul	21
7	Hepa-merz	13
8	Ademethionine	10
9	Antral	10
10	Sirepar	9
11	Liv-52.	8
12	Essel forte	8
13	Bonjigar	6
14	Lipoic acid	2
15	Hepatoritz	4
16	Fosfogliv	1
17	Rezalut	1
18	Sibectan	1
Total:		**534**

Out of 36 names of the studied hepatoprotectors 18 were not used by patients at all. The used hepatoprotectors were used separately and in combination. In 6,9% (15 patients) out of 239 patients no hepatoprotectors were used, 23,4% (56 patients) - one hepatoprotector was recommended, among them the most frequently used were essential phospholipids and UDCA, 29,7% (71 patients) - combination of two drugs, the most frequent combination was essential phospholipids-riboxin, 26,4% (63 patients) - combination of three drugs, the most frequent combination was essential phospholipids-riboxin-carsyl, 13.0% (31 patients) - four drugs were combined, the most frequent combination was essential phospholipids-riboxin- thiotriosalin-UDHC, 1.3% (3 patients) - five drugs were combined, the frequent combination was essential phospholipids-UDHC-riboxin-ademethionine- thiotriosalin.

When we studied the frequency of hepatoprotectors used during treatment, 18 types of hepatoprotectors were used 534 times in224 patients. Of them essential phospholipids were used in 161 patients - 1st place (30,2%), riboxin - 128 patients - 2nd place (24,0%), UDCA - 59 patients - 3rd place (11,1%), thiotriosaline - 54 patients - 4th place (10.1%), Karsil - 38 patients - 5th place (7.1%), Apcasul - 21 patients - 6th place (4.0%), Hepato-merz - 13 patients - 7th place (2.4%), ademetionine and antral - each to 10 patients - 8th place (1.9% each, 3.8% total), sirepar - 9 patients - 9th place (1.7%), liv-52 and essel-forte - each to 8 patients - 10th place (1.5% each, 3,0%), bonjigar - 6 patients - 11th place (1.1%), lipoic acid - 2 patients - 12th place (0.4%), drugs phosphogliv, resalut, sibectan - 13th place - each for 1 patient (0.2% each, 0.6% in total).

As noted above, 18 out of 36 names of the studied hepatoprotectors were not used at all during inpatient treatment, and the other 18 were used successfully: 214 (89.5%) out of 239 treated patients improved their general condition, and 16 (6.7%) had practically no changes, 5 (2.1%) worsened their general condition, and 4 (1.7%) died. The analysis of patients' medical records showed that the worsening of their condition and the occurrence of lethal outcomes were related not to the hepatoprotectors used, but to the extremely severe general condition of the patients.

When analysing the frequency of used hepatoprotectors by dosage forms, it was found that ampoules were the most frequently used, accounting for 70% of the total number of drugs used (Fig.). The lowest frequency was in vials, which accounted for 1.3%.

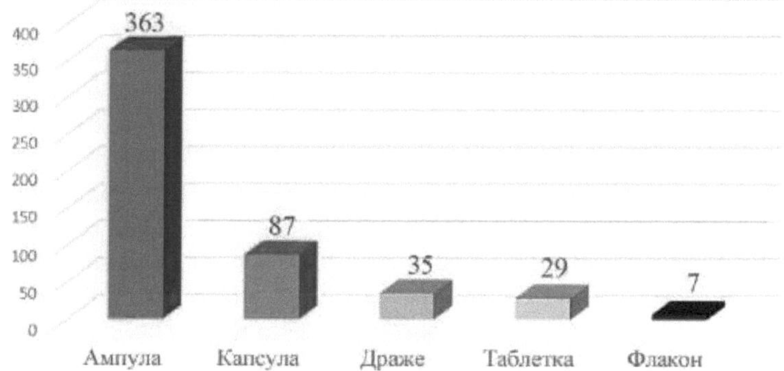

Frequency of dosage forms of hepatoprotectants used by patients with cirrhosis. by patients with liver cirrhosis.

The bulk of hepatoprotectors used were injectable forms, which accounted for 71.3% of the total frequency of hepatoprotectors used. Oral forms were used less frequently: capsules - 16.6%, dragees - 6.6%, tablets - 5.5%.

The data show that injectable hepatoprotectants are used more frequently than oral hepatoprotectants in the inpatient treatment of cirrhosis.

Based on the results obtained, it can be concluded that liver cirrhosis in terms of frequency of occurrence is higher in women than in men. The study of patients by age showed that it is more common in persons aged 40-60 years than in persons under 40 and over 60 years of age. This can be explained by the fact that the disease is asymptomatic in the early stages and patients are less likely to be diagnosed at an early stage due to late referral to a doctor, and it is less common in persons over 60 years of age, and it is possible to conclude that they often have a fatal outcome due to complications. And also, the number of patients living in urban areas is twice less than in rural areas, indicating that the rural population has low medical culture or low self-esteem compared to the urban population and therefore rarely seek medical help. In the vast majority of these patients, the disease lasted from 5 to 10 years or more. Among the drugs used in their treatment, the main place was occupied by hepatoprotectors, which accounted for an average of 2.4 hepatoprotectors per patient. The next place was occupied by vitamins, drugs affecting water and salt metabolism, and diuretics. The level of use of the other groups was very low.

Of the 36 studied hepatoprotectors, 18 were not used by patients at all, and the other 18 were used 534 times individually and in combination. At the same time, essential phospholipids, riboxin, UDCA and thiotriosalin, each of the drugs, were used in more than 10% of patients, and the frequency of use of other hepatoprotectors did not reach 10%.

During the study period, it was found that an average of 6.4 different drugs were used per patient, including an average of 2.4 hepatoprotectants. It was found that the use of baseline drugs

in patients treated for cirrhosis was only 37.5%, and the remaining 62.3% were minor drugs. This suggests that good efficacy in the treatment of cirrhosis may not be achieved due to insufficient use of hepatotropic agents included in the standards of treatment of cirrhosis. However, despite this, the overall condition of 89.5 per cent of patients treated in regional health facilities improved. Most of the hepatoprotectors used were injectable, accounting for 71.3% of the total number of hepatoprotectors used. This confirmed the idea that patients with liver cirrhosis should be administered parenterally due to a significant decrease in absorption in the gastrointestinal tract.

Comparing the obtained results with the data of previous studies, we see that in Bukhara and Navoi oblasts during inpatient treatment of hepatobiliary system diseases essential phospholipid preparations and Karsil were used mainly in injectable form in more than 80% of cases, in Khorezm oblast essential phospholipids were used mainly in the treatment of liver cirrhosis 54% in most cases effectively used in injectable form. The use of UDCC was only 5% in Bukhara and Navoi oblasts and 11% in Khorezm oblast.

Thus, in Bukhara and Navoi oblasts essential phospholipids and Karsil were widely used as the main treatment in patients with hepatobiliary system diseases, and in Khorezm oblast essential phospholipids and riboxin were widely used in the treatment of liver cirrhosis. "Pharmacoeconomic analysis of hepatoprotectors used in patients with liver cirrhosis in some treatment and prevention institutions of Khorezm region", it also analysed the cost of treatment of patients with liver cirrhosis using ABC/VEN analyses as a pharmacoeconomic analysis.

The case histories of patients treated with diseases of hepatobiliary system and liver cirrhosis in regional hospitals from 2006 to 2013 were selected for retrospective study, information on drugs purchased by Khorezm region "Dori-Darmon" JSC from the state budget for treatment and preventive care institutions was provided from all state budgets of the region for the period from 2012 to 2016. ABC/VEN analyses of pharmacotherapy performed in patients treated in these years were carried out in more detail on the case histories of patients treated as inpatients in the treatment and prevention facilities of the region in 2013, as well as on the basis of information on drugs purchased from the state budget for treatment and prevention facilities of "Dori Darmon" JSC in the Khorezm region, provided by all state budgets of the region.

ABC-analysis of some characteristics of medicines purchased by JSC "Dori-Darmon" of Khorezm region in 2013 at the expense of the state budget of medical and preventive institutions provided from all state budgets of the region was as follows (Table).

ABC-analysis of drugs received by JSC "Dori-Darmon" of Khorezm region for 2013 during procurement at the expense of the state budget

groups	Funds spent on medicines (percentage)	Number of medicines	
		By. titles	Percentage
A	79	16	14,0
B	15	30	25,0
C	6	72	61,0
Total:	100	118	100

A total of 118 items of various medicines were procured during the year for the amount of UZS 3,363,158,522.73 (three billion three hundred sixty-three million one hundred fifty-eight thousand five hundred twenty-two UZS 73 tyiin). Of these, 2,668,593,723.88 (two billion six hundred sixty-eight million five hundred ninety-three thousand seven hundred twenty-three UZS 88 tyiin) medicines belonging to group A of 16 items and accounted for 79.0 per cent of the total expenditure. Medicines belonging to group B of 30 items totalled UZS 502,717,865.37 (five hundred two million seven hundred seventeen thousand eight hundred sixty-five thousand UZS 37 tiyin), which accounted for 15.0% of the total cost. Medicines belonging to group C of 72 items make up the amount of 191,846,933.48 soums (one hundred ninety one million eight hundred forty six thousand nine hundred thirty three soums 48tiyin), which is 6.0% of the total cost.

VEN analysis (Table) of these drugs was conducted in relation to the hepatobiliary system diseases we studied. The results of the analysis are as follows: category V, i.e. essential drugs, comprised 14 out of 118 items, representing 12% and 6% of the total expenditure, i.e. 200,820,406.49 (two hundred million eight hundred and twenty thousand four hundred and six soums 49 tiyin). Category E, i.e. drugs of high necessity but not absolute, comprised 55 items, accounting for 46.5% and 53% of the total expenditure on them, i.e. 1,788,844,145.32 (one billion seven hundred and eighty-eight million eight hundred and forty-four thousand one hundred and forty-five soums 32 tiyin) soums. Category N, i.e. drugs of doubtful value, includes 49 items, which is 41.5 per cent and 41 per cent of the total expenditure on them, i.e. 1,373,493,970.92 (one billion three hundred and seventy-three million four hundred and ninety-three thousand nine hundred and seventy-three thousand one hundred and seventy-five sums 92 tiyin) UZS.

VEN-analysis of drugs received in the procurement of "Dori Darmon" JSC Khorezm region in 2013 at the expense of the state budget

Category	Amount of drug in each category (percentage)	Percentage of funds spent on each category (percentage)
V	12	6
E	46,5	53
N	41,5	41

ABC-analysis of pharmacotherapeutic agents used for inpatient treatment of patients with liver cirrhosis in some hospitals of Khorezm region was as follows (Table). Medicines belonging to group A of 8 items totalled 1,848,122.48 (one million eight hundred forty-eight thousand one hundred twelve sums 48 tiyin) sums, which was 80.5% of the total cost. Medicines belonging to group B of 16 items totalled 347,009.99 soums (three hundred forty seven thousand nine soums 99 tiyin) and accounted for 15.0% of the total cost. Medicines belonging to group C of 20 items totalled 99,951.98 soums (ninety nine thousand nine hundred and fifty one soums 98 tiyin), which accounted for 4.5% of the total cost.

The results of VEN-analysis of pharmacotherapy (Fig. 2) in inpatients cured of liver cirrhosis in some hospitals of the region were as follows: Category V, i.e. vital drugs from 11 items, the total amount of which was 1,353,492.31 (one million three hundred and fifty-three thousand four hundred and ninety-two soum 31tiyin). Category E, i.e. high necessity drugs of 18 items, the total amount of which was 750,040.75 (seven hundred and fifty thousand forty rubles 75 tiyin). Category N, i.e. preparations of doubtful importance out of 15 items, the total amount of which amounted to 191,541.39 (one hundred and ninety-one thousand five hundred and forty-one sum 39 tiyin).

PWA analysis of used pharmacotherapeutic agents by patients hospitalised with liver cirrhosis in inpatient departments of some hospitals in Khorezm region in 2013.

groups	Expenditure on medicines (percentage)	Number of medicines	
		According to the name	Percentage
A	80,5	8	18
B	15,0	16	36
C	4,5	20	46
Bottom line:	100	44	100

From the above data, 25% or 11 out of 44 drugs used in pharmacotherapy of inpatients with liver cirrhosis in some hospitals of Khorezm region in 2013 belonged to category V, which accounted for 59% of the total expenditure, 41% or 18 items out of the total number of drugs used belonged to category E, which corresponds to 33% of the total expenditure, 34% of the total number of drugs used out of 15 items belonged to category N, which corresponds to 8% of the total cost of funds spent, can be explained by the fact that the liver cirrhosis inpatients in Khorezm region in 2013 belonged to category V, which accounted for 59% of the total cost of funds spent.

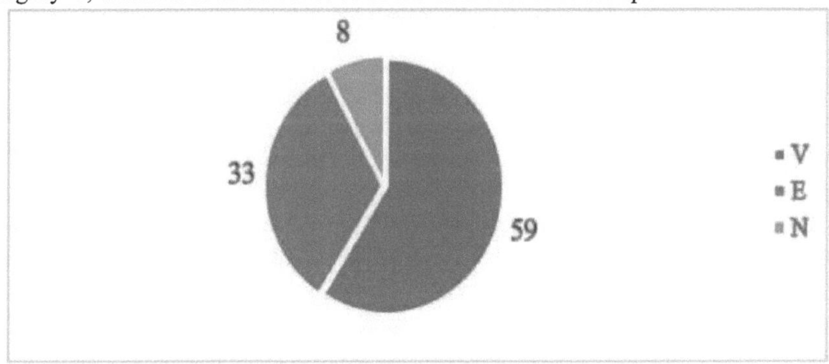

Results of a VEN analysis of pharmacotherapy in patients hospitalised with cirrhosis in some hospitals Khorezm region in 2013, as a percentage of total costs for the year.

Thus, according to the results of ABC/VEN-analyses, it can be seen that the funds spent on the studied LHUs at the regional level were used rationally, as 2/3 of drugs in group A belong to category V, almost 1/3 to category E and a minimal amount to category N. At the same time, ABC-analysis of expenditures on drugs used in inpatients with cirrhosis in the region showed that the most expensive drugs in group A are hepatoprotectors, followed by metabolic agents.

Comparing the results of ABC/VEN-analyses with the results of other scientific studies, the following picture emerged: in Bukhara and Navoi oblasts ABC-analysis of

drugs used in patients under inpatient treatment with hepatobiliary system disease showed that the most expensive drugs (group A) were infusion solutions and metabolic drugs, but in this group the share of hepatoprotectors was insufficient. According to the results of pharmacoeconomic analysis of pharmacotherapeutic agents data (ABC/VEN analyses), one quarter were the most expensive drugs (group A), the second most expensive were infusion solutions and metabolic agents (category N).
At the same time, a total of 11 types of hepatoprotectors used in the analysis of pharmacotherapy in inpatients with cirrhosis in Khiva and Khanka district medical centres in 2013 amounted to 1,353,492.31 (one million three hundred fifty-three thousand four hundred ninety-two UZS 31 tiyin). If we examine this amount for each type of hepatoprotector, we can see that the largest amount of money was spent on ademetionine and baseline drugs, which accounted for 35.4% and 32.3% of the amount, respectively. This means that the amount spent on these two drugs accounted for more than 60% of the total cost. According to the table, it was found that the relatively less expensive drugs were thiocetam, UDCC, thiotriosaline and hepatoric, while the least expensive drugs were Resolute, Carsil, Apcosul, Antral and Riboxin.
Also, 2,295,074.45 (two million two hundred ninety-five thousand seventy-four sums 45 tiyin) soums were spent on treatment of 16 patients with liver cirrhosis in the region during the year, on average 143,442.15 (one thousand four hundred forty-two sums 15 tiyin) soums per patient, but this amount did not include the drugs used as etiotropic treatment.
It is reliable that in the process of analysing the obtained results, we again found it necessary to pay special attention to the following. In particular, in 2013 JSC "Khorezm Dori Darmon" purchased 14 types of hepatoprotectors at the expense of the state budget in the amount of 200,820,406.49(two hundred million eight hundred twenty-four thousand six hundred and 49 tiyin) soum. However, in 2013, 11 types of hepatoprotectors for inpatients with liver cirrhosis were used in Khiva and Khanka district medical associations, including 7 types of hepatoprotectors worth 787,908.47 (seven hundred and eighty seven thousand nine hundred and eighty eight sums 47 tiyin) sums and 565,583.84 (five hundred and sixty five thousand five hundred and eighty three sums 84 tiyin) sums, hepatoprotectors of the remaining 4 items were purchased at the expense of patients' own funds. Thus, instead of effectively using 14 types of hepatoprotectors purchased by Khorezm Dori Darmon JSC at the expense of the state budget, patients purchased other types of hepatoprotectors at their own expense.
Thus, the results of ABC/VEN analyses showed that state financial resources allocated for hepatoprotectors, which are not included in the standards of liver cirrhosis treatment, were spent in larger amounts and used irrationally. In all the hospitals studied, 4/5 of the medicines used for inpatient treatment were purchased at public expense, and 1/5 at the patients' own expense. The average cost per patient treated for liver cirrhosis in the region for the year was 143,442.15 (one hundred and forty-three thousand four hundred and forty-two sums 15 tiyin), but this amount did not include

drugs used as etiotropic treatment. Based on the above, we developed a "Local Drug Formulary" based on the analysis of selection and evaluation of the effectiveness of hepatoprotectors in the treatment of liver cirrhosis in the Khorezm region, which showed the lack of a unified approach and pharmacoeconomic basis for their use by doctors of different specialities and implemented in practice.

1. It was found that in the whole region each patient with liver cirrhosis corresponds to an average of 6.4 names of used medicines, per patient - 3, 4 and even 5 names of hepatoprotectors were used simultaneously in combination with each other and polyprogmasia was allowed. Physicians did not identify the aetiological factors and did not apply the appropriate
etiotropic treatment.
2. It was found that in Khiva and Khanka districts essential phospholipids and riboxin were widely used as basic therapeutic agents in the treatment of patients with liver cirrhosis, and in Khorezm Regional Multidisciplinary Medical Centre - ademetionine and UDCA.
3. Based on the results of ABC/VEN analyses, it was found that state financial resources allocated for hepatoprotectants not included in the standards of liver cirrhosis treatment were spent in large quantities and used irrationally. In all studied hospitals, 4/5 of the pharmacotherapeutic agents used for inpatient treatment were purchased at the expense of the state, and 1/5 - at the expense of patients' own funds.
4. It was determined that the average cost per patient treated for liver cirrhosis in the region for the year was 143,442.15 (one hundred forty-three thousand four hundred forty-two UZS 15 tiyin) UZS, but this amount did not include drugs used as etiotropic treatment.
5. The "Local Drug Formulary" was developed and introduced into practice on the basis of the analysis of selection and evaluation of the effectiveness of hepatoprotectors in the treatment of liver cirrhosis in the Khorezm region, which showed the lack of a unified approach and pharmacoeconomic basis for their use by doctors of different specialities.

Also in the study "Modern ideas about congenital heart defects in children" conducted in our branch the results of analysis of modern scientific researches devoted to etiopathogenesis and classification of congenital heart defects, their prevalence taking into account different climatogeographical conditions, laboratory markers of myocardial adaptation in CHD in children, as well as the importance of physical rehabilitation of children with congenital heart defects are presented.

A prospective cohort study was conducted for 108 children diagnosed with CHD aged 1 to 13 years (mean age - 7.84±0.8 years) between 2019 and 2022. Clinical material was collected at the multidisciplinary polyclinic of the urban settlement of Khanki, Khorezm region. Laboratory and instrumental studies were conducted at the Republican Specialised Scientific and Practical Centre of Cardiology and Cardiac Surgery of the Aral Sea region and the regional children's hospital.

In the main group of children, subgroups were formed depending on the severity of

CHF and functional class (FC): Group 1 - 55 children with CHS-0, Group 2 - 28 children with IΦK CHS I degree, Group 3 - 25 children with IIΦK CHS IIA degree. The age distribution of the examined children is presented in the table below

Distribution of children by age in the study groups

Study groups	1-3 years Abs/%/ cf. Age	4-6 lees Abs/%/. middle age	7-13 ages Abs/%/. middle age
1 - group Children without CHF, n=55	8/14,5/ 1,44±0,16	11/ 20/ 4,99±0,32	36/ 65,5/ 9,52±0,31
2 - group Children with CHF stage I (SC) n=28	8/ 28,6/ 1,77±0,36	7/ 25/ 5,18±0,31	13/ 46,4/ 9,77±0,62
3 -group Children with CHF stage IIA (PFC) n=25	7/ 28,0/ 1,54±0,34	8/ 32,0/ 5,41±0,32	10/ 40,0/ 9,81±0,50
Total children with CHD, n=108	23/ 21,3	26/ 24,1	59/ 54,6
Control group, n=40	8/ 20 1,52±0,21	11/ 27,5 5,0±0,40	21/ 52,5 9,70±0,42

The severity of CHF was determined on the basis of complaints, anamnestic data and physical examination, according to the ACC/AHA (American Society of Cardiology/American Heart Association) classification. This classification is similar to the classification of Vasilenko V.H. and Strajesko N.D. and was used in children of preschool and school age. CSF AC was diagnosed according to the NYHA classification (New York Heart Association). For children of early age the stages of CHF taking into account clinical criteria were determined in accordance with the classification of Belokon N.A. (1978). FC in children of early and preschool age - according to the classification of Ross (2016). The control group of the study consisted of 40 practically healthy children (I - II health groups according to M.S. Grombach, 1982, with additions, 2003) of similar age (mean age - 6.6±0.42 years).
Inclusion criteria in the main group were: age of children from 1 year to 13 years with established diagnosis of CHD, condition after surgical correction of CHD, with CHD-0, IΦK CHD I and IIΦK CHD IIA stage, parental consent for the study. Exclusion criteria were as follows: age of children younger than 1 year and older than 13 years, condition after surgical correction of CHD with CHD IIE and III stages, children from multiple pregnancies, children born with very low and extremely low body weight, children with extracardiac pathology in the decompensation stage, parents' refusal to participate in the study.
The clinical diagnosis of CHD was established in accordance with the generally accepted classification based on the clinical and instrumental picture of the disease. The most frequent septal malformations were registered in 77.2% (85) of cases. In terms of the frequency of occurrence, the first place was occupied by the PAD (65.4%

(72)). Pulmonary artery stenosis was observed in 5.45% of cases, triad and Fallot's tetrad in 4 (3.64%) children. Open ductus arteriosus, common atrioventricular canal (complete and incomplete types) occurred in 10.0% of cases. We performed complex investigations using standard methods: questionnaire survey, ante- and postnatal anamnesis; clinical examination included BP measurement, anthropometry according to WHO criteria (2,009); ultrasound examination of the thyroid gland, kidneys, abdominal and pelvic organs was performed according to generally accepted standards on a Chison Cbit8 ultrasound diagnostic system.

Laboratory investigation was carried out in the clinical and biochemical laboratory of RSNPC of Cardiology and Cardiac Surgery of the Aral Sea region and included: general blood analysis, general urine analysis, hepatic transaminases, determination of the level of high-sensitivity C-reactive protein (CR Phs), troponin I (cTnI) and N-terminal pro-brain natriuretic peptide (NT- pro BNP). Concentrations of CRP-hs, cTnI and NT- proBNP in blood serum were determined by immunochemical method on Finecare analyser by Wondfo company (manufacturer - People's Republic of China).

A comparative analysis of morphometric and haemodynamic parameters according to echocardiographic data was carried out with those of healthy children depending on body surface area (Klaidaiter U. et al., 2022). Echocardiographic parameters were studied. Ultrasound duplex scanning of the common carotid arteries on a Sonospape SSI-500 ultrasound scanner, Mindray (Holland), was performed to assess vascular haemodynamic parameters. The adaptation potential index (API) of the cardiovascular system (CVS) of R.M.Baevsky et al. (1987) was calculated. The index value below 2.6 points was interpreted as satisfactory adaptation, 2.6-3.09 points - tension of adaptation mechanisms, 3.10-3.49 - unsatisfactory adaptation and over 3.5 points - adaptation failure.

The programme of cardiac rehabilitation measures included non-medication therapy: nutrition adequate to physiological needs, therapeutic massage, therapeutic gymnastics. In addition, training seminars were held for parents to improve the effectiveness of cardiac rehabilitation measures. Children were under the supervision of a family physician, a cardiac surgeon, a neurologist and a physiotherapist. The effectiveness of cardiac rehabilitation measures was assessed by monitoring HR, BP, Martinet-Kushelevsky and Stange tests, electro- and echocardiography, as well as laboratory parameters: levels of high-sensitivity troponin I and brain natriuretic peptide NT-proBNP.

For the period from2019 to 2021, 110 children diagnosed with CHD were registered in the multidisciplinary polyclinic of the urban settlement of Khanki, Khorezm region (in 2019 - 32, in 2020 - 25, in 2021 - 53 children). 59.1% of children were taken into account at the primary preventive examination, the remaining 40.9% went to the polyclinic for the purpose of dynamic examination and/or treatment of somatic pathology and the diagnosis of CHD was a diagnostic finding. It was found that the incidence of CHD among boys was greater than in girls was 1.3:1 in 2019; 1.6:1-2020;1.5:1 in 2021. In the structure of CHD, interventricular septal defect ranked first

(65.4%), interatrial septal defect (11.8%) and OAP ranked second and third, OAK were 10.0% and pulmonary artery stenosis was 5.45%.

In most cases, CHD was diagnosed before the age of 1 year (45/40.9%) and surgical correction was performed in 11.8% (13) of cases. In 22.7% of cases, CHD occurred without clinical manifestations of circulatory disorders, which may be a possible reason for late presentation and untimely diagnosis of this disease. In the neonatal period, CHD was detected in 15 children (13.6%) and surgical care was provided only in 4.5% (5) of cases. CHD was diagnosed in 13 children (11.8%) in the third year of life and over three years of age in 37 (33.7%) children. (Figure 1). In 55 (50.9%) children no CHD was observed, which indicates the disappearance of haemodynamic disorders after cardiac surgical correction of CHD in 50.9% of cases. In the Russian Federation, these indicators are much higher: according to Baranov A.A. et al. (2016), positive dynamics after surgical intervention is found in 78% of cases.

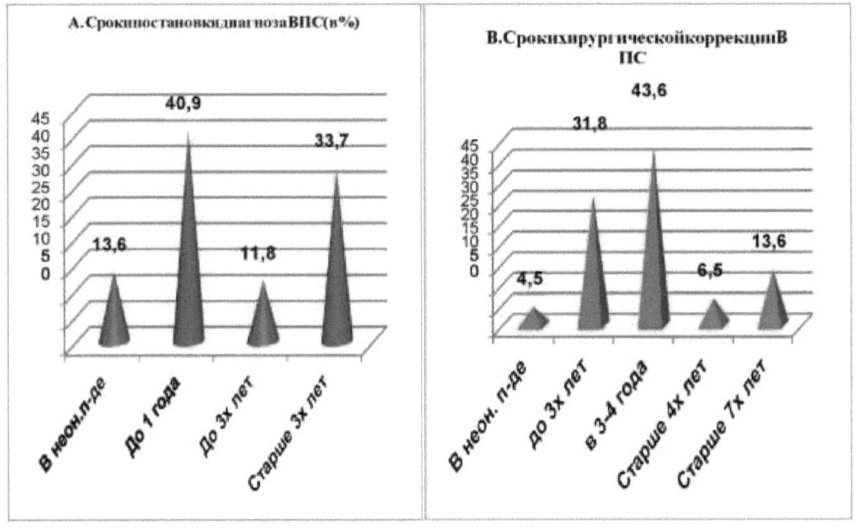

Figure 1. Timing of diagnosis (A) and surgical correction (B) of the examined children with CHD

During the analysis of anamnestic data of mothers of children born with congenital heart defects, the causes that could influence the formation of anatomical disorder of heart structures in the intrauterine period were identified. According to the results of logistic regression analysis, the most significant risk factors for CHD were: iron deficiency anaemia (OR=7.81, $p<0.001$), ARVI in the first trimester of pregnancy (OR=4.37, $p<0.01$), threat of pregnancy termination (OR=3.74, $p<0.01$), fetoplacental insufficiency (OR=3.46, $p<0.01$).

"Specific markers of myocardial adaptation in congenital heart disease in children: levels of NT-proBNP and troponin I in correlation with C-reactive protein" presents the results of analyses of relationships between the levels of specific markers of myocardial adaptation

NT-proBNP and troponin I and concentration of high-sensitivity C-reactive protein (CRPhs). The highest level of CRPhs was found in children with CHF IIA with a significant difference compared to the
control (p<0.001), group 1 (p<0.001) and group 2 (p<0.05). Significantly increased values of the level were also noted in children of group 2 (p<0.001) in relation to control and group 1 (p<0.001). In children of group 1, despite the absence of CHF, CRPhs values were significantly higher (p<0.001) than in controls (Table 2). For the group of children with CHF grade I, CRPhs level>5.2 mg/L had specificity (Sp=71%), sensitivity (Se=61.0%), relative risk RR=3.1, with reliable prognosis (Kass=0.60, p<0.01)

Average levels of CRPhs, NT-proBNP, cTnl in blood serum in the analysed groups

children in the analysed groups depending on age

groups	CRPhs, mg/l	NT-proBNP, ng/ml	cTnl,ng/ml
Control group, n=40			
1-3 years, n=8	0,51±0,7	142,3±8,7	0,01±0,005
4-6 years old, n=11	0,77±0,8	137,9±4,6	0,011±0,003
7-13 years old, n=21	1,2±0,6	159,7±3,2	0,012±0,001
Group 1, n=55			
1-3 years, n=8	4,2±0,8***	146,9±6,5	0,014±0,02
4-6 years old, n=11	4,4±0,7***	157,9±8,0*	0,012±0,01
7-13 years old, n=36	4,1±0,13***	163,7±2,9**	0,013±0,001
Group 2, n=28			
1-3 years, n=8	5,2±0,7***	286,7±18,4***л	0,16±0,03***
4-6 years old, n=7	6,0±0,9***	295.2±20.4***LLL	0,18±0,02**л
7-13 years old, n=13	6.2±0.6***L	300,4±24,0***	0.2±0.01***LLL
Group 3, n=25			
1-3 years, n=7	6,5±0,97***л	491.7±15.9***LLL####.	0,21±0,03**л
4-6 years old, n=8	7.1±0.85***L	548.2±18.2***LLL####.	0.24±0.02***LLL###.
7-13 years old, n=10	8e±1 1***LL	586.0±24.8***LLL####.	0.25±0.03***L

Note: * - p < 0.05; ** - p < 0.01; *** - p < 0.001 - reliability of differences between the values of indicators of the main groups of children with the control groups; LLL - p < 0.0010.001 - reliability of differences between the indicators of the 2nd and 3rd groups and the 1st group; - #- p < 0.05; ## - p < 0.01; ### - p < 0.001 - reliability of differences between the indicators of the 3rd group and the 2nd group.

A high level of association, concordance (K_{ass}=0.94, $p<0.001$, χ^2=28.4, $p<0.001$, RR=13.5), and therefore high sensitivity (S_e=88.2%) and specificity (S_p=80.3 were inherent in the factor -CRPhs <6.8 mg/L. At the same time, in % of cases positive test results allow correct diagnosis of CHF of the first degree in children.

Diagnostic levels of CR Phs >7.1 mg/L (K_{ass}=0.68, $p<0.01$, χ2=5.41, $p<0.05$, RR=3.3, Se=75%, Sp=64.1%) and CRPhs<9.3 mg/L (K_{ass}=0.88, $p<0.001$; χ^2=9.07, $p<0.01$; RR=9.0, S_e=90.0%, S_p=62.8%) characterised grade IIA CHD in children with CHD in the post-correction period with greater reliability.

The age analysis of NT-pro BNP values in children with CHD in the post-correction period showed that the highest values were observed in children aged 4-6 and 7-13 years of the 3rd group and were significantly higher than in the control (Table 2). The dynamics of NT- pro BNP values increase with age in each individual group with reliable differences was established.

Diagnostic levels of 268 ng/ml<XT-rhoBXR<327 ng/ml were significantly associated (K_{ass}=0.71, $p<0.01$; 0.92 $p<0.001$, χ^2=8.69, $p<0.01$; 22.9 $p<0.001$, respectively) and were associated with the presence of first-degree CHF. At the same time, the risk of formation of first-degree CHD increased from RR=4.6 to RR=11.6 times. NT-pro BNP 490nr/M4<NT-pro BNP 610 ng/ml, (K_{acc}=0.76, $p<0.01$; 0.82 $p<0.001$; χ^2=6.68, $p<0.01$; 9.69 $p<0.01$;

RR=5.14, RR=6.3, respectively) clearly characterised grade IIA CHF in children with corrected CHD.

There was a significant increase in the level of c TnI in children of groups 2 and 3 in relation to the control and group 1 (Table 2). Apparently, this is associated with the course of subacute myocardial ischaemia, as evidenced by abnormalities in the processes of repolarisation of ventricular myocardium according to ECG data. The level of troponin I (cTnI, ng/ml) in serum in children with CHD in the post-correction remote period in the age ranges from one year to 13 years has not been studied and requires further research with the development of normative values for children of these ages.

When assessing the serum troponin I (cTnI, ng/ml) level in the observed children depending on their age, a tendency for its values to increase with age was established. Children of groups 2 and 3 at the age of 7-13 years had the highest values than children aged 1-3 years or 4-6 years and had a significant difference with respect to the control and group 1 (Table).

Diagnostic troponin I levels of 0.13 ng/ml<eTn1<0.19ng/ml, were significantly associated and correlated (K_{ass}=0.89, $p<0.001$; 0.90, $p<0.001$, χ^2=25.2, $p<0.001$; 20.35, $p<0.001$, RR=8.16, 10.7; S e=80.0% and 85.7%, S_p=80.9% and 76.8%, respectively) (Table. 4). A diagnostic range of 0.21 ng/ml<sTn1<0.26ng/ml was reliably defined for CHF

Grade IIA for children with corrected CHD (K_{ass}=0.85, $p<0.001$; 0.92, $p<0.001$, χ^2=10.75, $p<0.001$; 14.1, $p<0.001$, RR=5.2 and 12.0; Se=81.2 and 69.0, respectively).

Thus, diagnostically significant levels of CRPhs (5.2Mr/4<CRPhs<6.8MrÁr and 7.1

Mr/4<CRPhs<9.3MrÁr), NT-pro BNP (268ng/ml<NT- proBNP<327nr/M4 and 490ng/ml< NT-pro BNP< 610 ng/ml) and cTnI, (0.13< NG/ML<CTN1<0.19NG/ML AND 0.21<NG/ML<CTN1<0.26NG/ML) characterising I, PFC and degrees of CHD, I and IIA, respectively, and the level of myocardial adaptation in children with corrected CHD.

In children of the 1st main group of all ages, the values of morphometric indices of the heart chambers correspond to Z - values -2SD +2SD standardised EchoCG indices according to PPT. The range of Z - values - 2SD and +2SD corresponds to normal values of the studied index (Klydaiter W. et al., 2022). But, in children of the 1st group at the age of 1 -3 years, the averaged indices of LV posterior wall thickness by 15% and left atrial dimensions (LAD) by 49.6% are reduced relative to the statistical average values. According to the principle of "functional antagonism" there is a strain of LV systolic activity by (fraction of decrease - FU=41,1±1,1%) hyperdynamic type (FU>38%). It is somewhat less pronounced in children in the age ranges of 4-6 and 7-12 years according to RLP: decrease of values by 18.8% and 16.6%, respectively. In the age ranges of 4-6 and 7-13 years, the right ventricular dimensions were increased by 35.4% and 62.5%, respectively, relative to the mean values. A similar trend can be traced quite naturally with respect to morphological indices of children of groups 2 and 3.

In children of the 2nd and 3rd groups at the age of 1-3 years, there is a significant increase in RRF values (p<0.001, p<0.001) relative to those of the control and 1st groups, respectively, as well as an increase in pulmonary trunk diameter (DLS, p<0.05 and p<0.001) - only relative to the control group and a decrease in FU (p<0.05, p<0.05) and PV (p<0.05) - relative to the 1st group in children of the 2nd group and the control group.0.05 and p<0.001) - only relative to the control group and decrease in FU (p<0.05), and PV (p<0.05) - relative to group 1 in group 2 children and to the control group in group 3 children (p<0.01, p<0.05, respectively) of this age (Fig.).

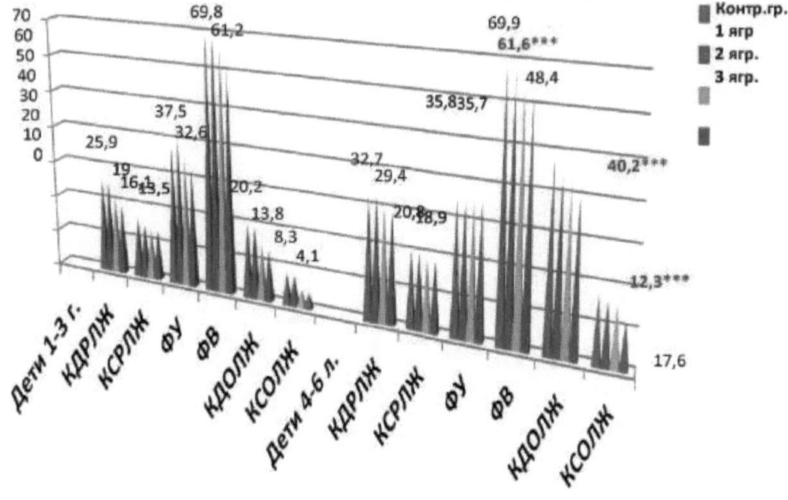

Fig. Main indices of systolic heart function in children aged 1-3 years and 4-6 years, analysed groups

An identical trend is observed in children in the age range of 4-6 years: a significant increase in RRF (p<0.001, p<0.001), DLs (p<0.01 and p<0.001) in the 2nd and 3rd groups of children in relation to the control and the 1st group. There was a significant decrease in EF (p<0.01, p<0.001) and LVEF (p<0.001, p<0.01), CSOLF (p<0.001, p<0.001), in relation to the control and the 1st group of this age.

A similar vector of development of morphometric capacities unfolds in the age range of children 7-13 years old. More pronounced reliable differences were established in relation to the indicators: decrease in LVADL (p<0.001, p<0.001), LVSDL (p<0.001, p<0.001), PV (p<0.01, p<0.001), increase in RRF (p<0.01, p<0.001) and DLs (p<<00.01 p<0.01 p<0.001), respectively, of children of groups 2 and 3, relative to the values of the control group and group 1 (Fig.).

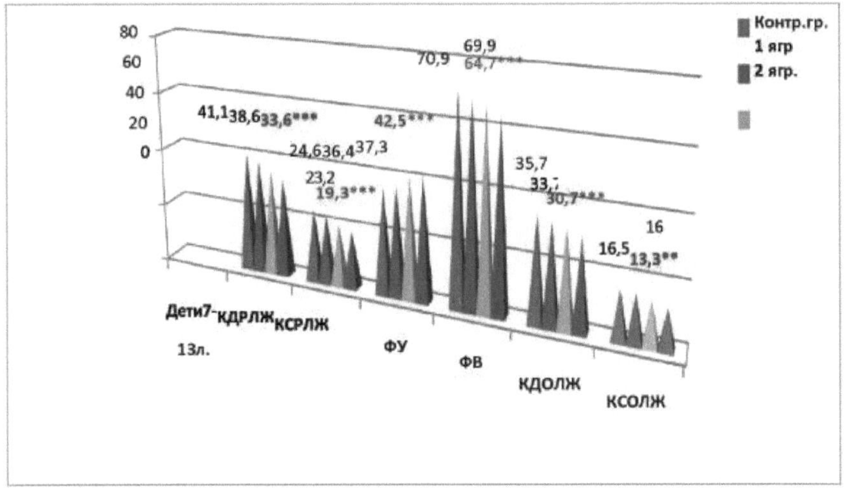

Main indices of systolic heart function in children aged 713 years, analysed groups

At this stage of myocardial structural and geometric myocardial remodelling, enlargement (dilation) of the LV and reduction of the LA are signs of diastolic dysfunction in the postoperative period. The most vulnerable in this respect were children of the 2nd and 3rd groups at the age of 1-3 years and 46 years, probably due to the short duration of the postoperative period and worse compensatory response.

Correlation analysis between morphometric values and indicators of physical development and haemoglobin and erythrocyte levels of the 1st group of children established close positive relationships (52 relationships): between CSFL and weight (r=0.67, p<0.01), height (r=0.57, p<0.05), protein-energy malnutrition of moderate degree (BENP) (r=0.72, p<0.001), almost identically between CSFL and weight (r=0.51, p<0.05), height (r=0.65, p<0.05), BENP0.05), BENP (r=0.81, p<0.001), between FVC and weight (r=-0.82, p<0.001), height (r=-0.82, p<0.001), BENP (r=-0.68, p<<0.05), BENP (r=-0.68, p<0.001)0.05) with a negative vector, between RLP and weight (r=0.78, p<0.001), height (r=0.86, p<0.001), BENP (r=0.79, p<0.001).

In children of group 2, correlation analysis showed the appearance of a close inverse relationship between RLF and weight (r=-0.57, p<0.05), height (r=-0.81, p<0.001), Hb level (r=-0.55, p<0.05). There were no associations between RLP and weight and height parameters, but significant interdependencies remained between RLP and weight (r=0.67, p<0.01), height (r=0.72, p<0.01), BENP (r=-0.57, p<0.05). Strong associations between DLs and weight (r=0.75, p<0.001), height (r=0.89, p<0.01), BENP (r=0.71, p<0.01), red blood cell count (r=0.94, p<0.001) were also recorded, which were absent in group 1.

In group 3 children, strong multidirectional correlations between RLP and weight (r=-0.98, p<0.001), height (r=-0.99, p<0.001), Hb level (r=0.89 p<0.001), red blood cell count (r=0.98, p<0.001) remained.0.001), there were also positive correlations between RLP and Hb level (r=0.68 p<0.01, erythrocyte count (r=0.72, p<0.01), which were negative in group 1 and absent in group 2.

Thus, in the mechanisms of regulation of morphometric indices of cardiac structures and, consequently, myocardial adaptation in children of group 1, optimal, regular pair correlations between morphometric values and clinical course of the postoperative period with the absence of CHF are traced. In groups of children with IOK CHF I and PFC CHF IIA degree reliable pair correlations between morphometric values and indicators of physical development, haemoglobin level, erythrocyte count acquire different multidirectional dynamics of development.

Duplex scanning of extra- and intracranial sections of brachiocephalic arteries in children of control groups, depending on age, revealed physiological growth of the vessel lumen (diameter of OCA, VCA and NCA, mm) and, accordingly, a decrease in blood flow velocity (Vps, cm/s) and resistance index (RI), which is confirmed by literature data. Similar changes in the above parameters were found in children of group 1 in the age aspect without significant differences in relation to the control. It was found that in children of groups 2 and 3 the values of the diameter of the right OSA and its intra-extracranial branches tended to decrease in relation to the control without significant differences.

differences and only the index of NSA diameter (p<0,05) at 7-13 years of age in children of the 3rd group was significantly low relative to the control (Fig.).

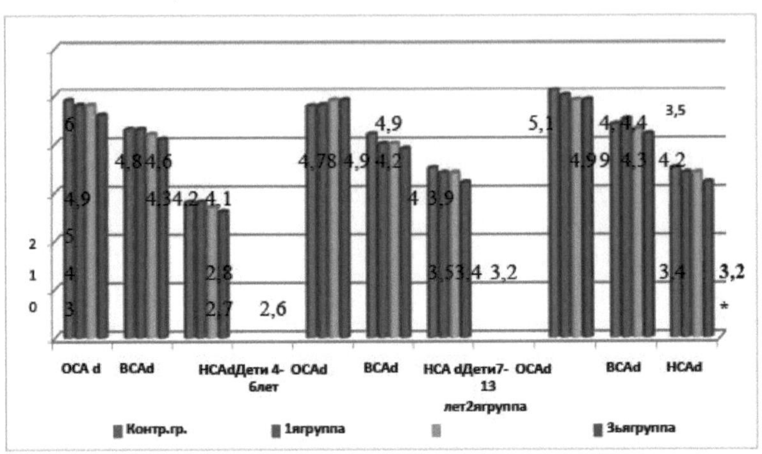

Mean values of diameters of OSA, VCA and NCA of children in the analysed groups

groups depending on age

Only blood flow velocity in the NCA (HCAVps, $p<0.001$) in children 4-6 years old of group 3 was significantly different relative to the control (Fig.6). At the age of 7-13 years, children of groups 2 and 3 had low values of OCA, VCA and NCA diameters and significantly increased blood flow velocity indices (OCAVps, $p<0.05$; BCAVps, $p<0.05$; HCAVps, $p<0.05$) in children of group 3 relative to control with high RI values on OCA, VCA and NCA, with no significant differences.

The TCIM study makes it possible to assess the risk of medium- and long-term complications in the postoperative period in children with CHD. According to the results of our study, in children of the 3rd group, the mean value of OSA TCIM was 9.2%, 12.5% and 10.3% higher in children in the age ranges 1-3 years, 4-6 years and 7-13 years, respectively, than in controls.

Thus, duplex examination of the common carotid artery and its branches is a convenient and reliable method of early detection of arterial lesions as target organs in children for the development of cephalgic complications in the mid- and long-term in the postoperative period in children with CHD with CHD stage I and IIA. The study showed that at 4-6 years of age, the presence of stage I CHD increases the risk of impaired velocity haemodynamic parameters by 3.5 ($K_{ass}=0.84$, $p<0.001$) times, and in CCN IIA - by 7.7 ($K_{ass}=0.94$, $p<0.001$) times, in 7-13 years - by 7.5 ($K_{(ass)}=0.92$, $p<0.001$) and 25 ($K_{ass}=0.97$, $p<0.001$) times, respectively. Higher OSA TCIM values in children 7-13 years old in stage I CHF occur 5.6($K_{ass}=0.89$, $p<0.001$) times, and 14.6 times in stage IIA CHF (K_{ass} =0,95, p<0,001)

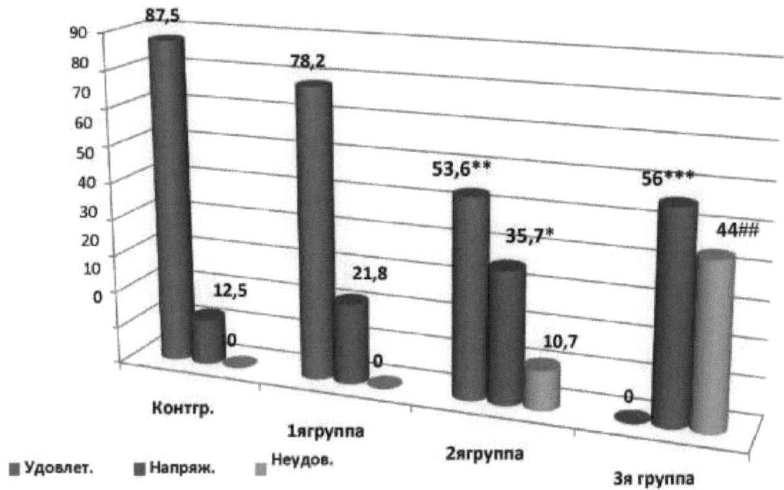

Note: * - p<0.05; ** - p<0.01; *** - p<0.001 - reliability of differences between the values of the main and control groups of children; ## - p<0.01 - reliability of differences between the values of the 2nd and 3rd groups of children

Frequency of occurrence of the levels of adaptation of the CCC in the analysed groups of children (in %)

For early diagnosis of myocardial adaptation disorders in children with congenital heart disease, the index of adaptation potential of the cardiovascular system (IAP) of R.M.Baevsky et al. (1987) was calculated in the analysed cohorts.

According to the presented data, the highest frequency of occurrence of SSS condition as "tension of adaptation mechanisms" was noted in the 3rd (p<0.001) and 2nd (p<0.05) groups in relation to the control.

"Unsatisfactory adaptation" of SSS was found only in the 2nd and 3rd (p<0.01) groups with a significant difference relative to the 2nd group. The average values of the AP index are presented in the table.

Averaged values of children's AP index depending on the presence/absence of CVD (in points)

groups	Satisfactory adaptation	Voltage mech. Adaptation	Unsatisfied. adaptation
Control Group, n=40	2,2±0,01	2,7±0,01	-
Group 1, n=55	2,42±0,01	2,8±0,02***	-
Group 2, n=28	2,45±0,01	2.9±0.02***ΛΛΛ	3,16±0,02
Group 3, n=25	-	2.9±0.03***ΛΛ	3,32±0,03###

Note:***- p < 0.001 - p < 0.001 - reliability of differences between the values of the indicators of the main groups of children and the control group; $^{(\Lambda\Lambda)}$- p < 0.01, $^{\Lambda\Lambda\Lambda}$ - p

< 0.001 - reliability of differences between the indicators of the 2nd and 3rd groups and the 1st group; ### - p < 0.001 - reliability of differences between the indicators of the 3rd group and the 2nd group.

Significant differences in the values of "tension of adaptation mechanisms" in the main groups (p<0.001, respectively for groups 1, 2 and 3) were found relative to the control. In the presence of CHF, the analysed values of groups 2 and 3 were significantly higher (p<0.001, p<0.01, respectively) than in group 1 of children with CHF-0. Unsatisfactory adaptation was found only in the 2nd and 3rd groups of children. Reliably high average values of IAP (p<0.001) were found in children of group 3, relative to group 2.

The AP index value <2.43 was significantly associated (K_{ass}=0.99, p<0.001, χ^2 = 2.31, p<0.05, S_e=75%, S_p=45.6%) with satisfactory adaptation of SSc and clinically characterised by the absence of complaints in children, good health and absence of CHF. Despite this, children of group 1 had a 1.2-fold risk of adaptation mechanisms tension. Tension of adaptation mechanisms was characterised by IAP<2.92. This index had low sensitivity (S_e=66.7%) and specificity (S_p=65.6%), as it was more associated with IФK and CHF of the first degree (K_{ass}=0.55, p<0.05, χ^2 4.03, p<0.05) with a risk of its development in (RR=2.24) 2.24 times. In clinical condition: children well tolerated habitual physical activity, which was not accompanied by rapid fatigue, dyspnoea or palpitations, moderate degree of BENP, high normal CAD relative to the child's height, sinus tachyarrhythmia and incomplete blockade of the right leg of the Gis bundle on electrocardiogram were revealed.

A reliable relationship between CRPhs, NT-proBNP levels and AP index (r=0,66, p<0,01, r=0,83, p<0,001, respectively) in the group of children with IФK and CHF of the 1st degree was established. In control (r=0,41, p>0,05) and 1st main (r=0,34, p>0,05 and r=0,03, p>0,1) groups of children the described similar reliable correlation was absent.

Unsatisfactory adaptation with AP index <3.18 was more often registered in group 3 children with CHF IIA degree and PFC. There was a slight limitation of physical activity: at rest there were no symptoms, habitual physical activity was accompanied by fatigue, dyspnoea or palpitations. Moderate BENP and disharmonious physical development were prevalent in the children. This range of IAPs had a significant association coefficient (K_{ass}=0.87, p<0.001, χ^2 = 7.53, p<0.01), good sensitivity (S_e=78.6%) but low specificity (S_p=64.1%). Direct strong correlations were found between IIA degree of CHF (r=0.82, p<0.001), NT-proBNP levels (r=0.93, p<0.001), cTnI (r=0.74, p<0.01) and the frequency of "unsatisfactory" adaptation profile of group 3 children with corrected CHD.

For early diagnosis of myocardial adaptation we have developed reliable diagnostic ranges of morphometric indicators of echocardiography and specific markers of myocardial adaptation (levels of NT-proBNP and troponin I in correlation with C-reactive protein) by age and three levels of adaptation potential (tabl).

Diagnostic criteria of myocardial adaptation in children with

Congenital heart defects in the postoperative period

Indicators	Levels of myocardial adaptation		
	Satisfactory. adaptation	Tension of adaptation mechanisms	Unsatisfactory d. adaptation
CRPhs (mg/litre)	<5,0	5,2 - 6,8	7,1 - 9,3
NT-proBNP (ng/ml)	<150,2	268 -327	490 -610
cTnl (ng/ml)	<0,13	0,13 -0,19	0,21 - 0,26
Echocardiogram: PV (%) 1-3 years	>65,7	<65,6	<63,4
Ages 4-6	>69,1	<69,0	<65,0
7-13 years old	>69,5	<69,4	<65,6
KDOLJ (ml) 1-3 d.	>19,8	<19,7	<13,8
Ages 4-6	>47,0	<46,9	<40,2
7-13 years old	>34,1	<34,0	<30,7
CSOLJ (ml) 1-3 d.	>7,3	<7,2	<5,0
Ages 4-6	>13,6	<13,5	<12,6
7-13 years old	>16,2	<16,1	<13,3
RPW (mm) 1-3 yr.	<10,6	>10,7	>20,5
Ages 4-6	<14,3	>14,4	>22,5
7-13 years old	<15,6	>15,7	>26,4
RLP (mm) 1-3 yr.	>17,8	<17,7	<16,1
Ages 4-6	>20,0	<19,9	<16,5
7-13 years old	>22,0	<21,9	<17,2
DLS (mm) 1-3 years	<16,2	>16,3	>21,6
Ages 4-6	<19,0	>19,1	>25,4
7-13 years old	<21,9	>22,0	>28,3
IAP (points)	<2,43	<2,92	<3,18

Tension of adaptation mechanisms by FV was in the range of 65.7%<FV<69.4% (Kass=0.92, p<0.001, χ^2=28.1, p<0.001, RR=11.4, Se=84.0%, Sp=81.0%).

The range of FV 61.2%<FV<65.6% was associated (Kass=0.97, p<0.001, χ^2=46.6, p<0.001, Se=86.9%, Sp=91.2%) with a poor state of myocardial adaptation with a 16-fold relative risk of developing its dysfunction (RR=16.0) and corresponded to IIΦK CHS grade IIA.

The examined children were divided into 2 groups, each of which was divided into 2 subgroups: 1st main group - 7 children aged 4-6 years with !FC of CCN I degree; 2nd main group - 12 children aged 7-13 years with IΦK CCN I; comparison groups: Group 3 - 11 children aged 4-6 years without CCN and Group 4 - 20 children aged 7-13 years without CCN. The duration of the postoperative period was 2.5 ± 1.4 years in the first group and 3.4 ± 1.8 years in the second group.

The results were evaluated in the 4 groups after 12 months, with repeated paraclinical

examinations.
In the main and comparison groups, interventions were designed and implemented for each child individually, taking into account BMI, dietary preferences and physical fitness.
Analysis of the initial averaged values of the Martinet-Kushelevsky test revealed that HR and BP after exercise statistically significantly increased in children of all four groups, and their full recovery occurred after 5 minutes. All the examined children had a hypertensive type of cardiovascular system response to physical exercise: there was a more pronounced increase in HR almost 1.5 times, the increase in CAD was 69.3%, as well as an increase in MAP by 12.4% of the initial one. In addition, there was a significant increase in HR at the 1st minute with a significant difference in children of the 1st ($p < 0.05$) and 2nd ($p < 0.05$) main groups in relation to the comparative group. Slowdown of recovery time was revealed - more than 7 minutes and had a significant difference between groups (1st, $p < 0.05$ and 2nd, $p < 0.05$, groups, relative to the groups of comparison, respectively).
The increase in both systolic and diastolic BP after exercise was also characterised by more significantly higher values in children of the main group at the 1st (group 1 CAD and MAP $p<0.05$ and group 2 $p<0.05$, respectively, relative to the comparison groups) and 3rd minute (group 1 CAD and MAP $p<0.05$ and group 2 $p<0.05$, respectively, relative to the comparison groups).0,05, $p<0,05$ and 2nd group $p<0,05$, $p<0,05$, respectively relative to the comparison groups) and at the 3rd minute (CAD and DAD of the 1st group $p<0,05$, $p<0,05$ and 2nd group $p<0,05$, $p<0,05$, respectively relative to the comparison groups). Complete normalisation of CAD and DA in the recovery period occurred in children of the comparison groups, with a statistical difference in the values of CAD and DA in children of the main groups (group 1, $p<0.05$ and group 2, $p<0.05$), where complete normalisation was not registered. The special Stange respiratory test - breath-holding time after submaximal inhalation, showed a decrease in the results of the test in all examined children compared to the normative values with a significant difference only in the group of children aged 7-13 years.
The initial level of the damage marker high-sensitivity troponin I (c Tnl) had reliable statistical differences between groups and was 0.18±0.01 ng/ml ($p<0.001$) in group 1 and 0.19±0.01 ng/ml ($p<0.001$) in group 2 children versus group 3 (0.12±0.006 ng/ml) and group 4 (0.13±0.004 ng/ml). The numerical values of NT- pro BNP before rehabilitation measures also had significant statistical differences between groups and were 296.7±29.7 ng/ml in group 1 children versus 150.1±20.7 ng/ml in group 3 children ($p<0.001$), 293.5±23.4 ng/ml in group 2 and 4 children versus 147.1±15.5 ng/ml ($p<0.001$).
A control examination of 50 children after 12 months revealed that the majority of children in the main groups (94.7%) had improved their general condition, appetite, decreased fatigue, and increased physical activity as a result of the rehabilitation programme. A positive effect of the rehabilitation programme on anthropometric parameters compared to the initial indicators was noted. A reliable increase in BMI

frequency within +1CO and -1CO ($p<0.05$) was found in children aged 7-13 years, and in children aged 4-6 years - 2.5 times, with no significant differences.
The Martine-Kushelevsky test 12 months after the rehabilitation measures showed an improvement in all the studied parameters in children of the main groups, close to the data of the comparison groups. Thus, in children of the main groups the type of cardiovascular system response to physical exercise was normotonic: HR increased not more than 60% of the initial one, CAD not more than 30%, and MAP slightly decreased, which indicates an increase in cardiac output and a decrease in peripheral resistance. The result of the Stang test after 12 months in group 1 increased by 37.5%, and in group 2 - 32.8%.
Also in children of the main groups against the background of the complex of rehabilitation measures it was possible to achieve a decrease in the indices of myocardial damage marker - cTnl. Thus, the concentration of cTnl in blood serum in groups 1 and 2 decreased from 0.18 ± 0.01 to 0.13 ± 0.02 ng/ml, from 0.19 ± 0.01 to 0.15 ± 0.01 ng/ml, respectively. Analysis of the long-term follow-up results of 19 children after 12 months showed a significant ($p<0.05$) decrease in the heart failure biomarker NT-pro BNP in groups 1 and 2: from 296.7 ± 29.7 to 190.6 ± 32.2 ng/ml in group 1 ($p<0.05$) and to 168.4 ± 28.07 ng/ml in group 2 (vs 293.5 ± 23.4 ng/ml, $p<0.01$).
Thus, the results of the study showed that the developed complex of rehabilitation measures in the remote postoperative period in children with congenital heart disease contributed to normalisation of body mass index, improvement of general well-being, increase in physical endurance and tolerance to physical activity, as well as decrease in the activity of markers of myocardial damage and heart failure. It should also be noted that there were no hospitalisations in the groups of children who received complex rehabilitation for 12 months. The foregoing confirms the possibility and expediency of using this programme both in group and individual rehabilitation of children in the remote period after surgical correction of congenital heart disease.
Modern conceptions of Classification, epidemiology, etiopathogenesis of mastopathy, endocrinological aspects, in particular the influence of thyroid pathology on the breast and the advantages and disadvantages of diagnostic methods used in combination, the two pathologies were analysed and the aspects to be solved were identified. Laboratory charts of 184 patients treated with mastopathy and thyroid pathology from 2019 to 2021 at Urgench branch of Tashkent Medical Academy were obtained as the source of the study. Their laboratory data and ultrasound findings from outpatient charts and were subjected to dynamic monitoring for 3 years.
The patients underwent general clinical examination, objective and subjective examination (general examination, palpation of the thyroid and mammary glands, auscultation of the heart and vessels); instrumental investigations included ultrasound of the mammary glands and thyroid gland, mammography, electrocardiography (ECG) when indicated. Instrumental investigations included breast and thyroid ultrasound and mammography, fine-needle aspiration biopsy and its histological examination, thyroid scan, electrocardiogram examination as indicated. All patients were under observation

for 3 years, the above-mentioned examinations were observed in dynamics.
A fine-needle aspiration biopsy (TI-RADS) was obtained at ultrasound in patients with high categorisation in ACR TI-RADS and BIRADS.
Hormonal studies were performed using commercially available "MINDRAY 96A" enzyme-linked immunosorbent assay (ELISA) kits developed in China.
Thyroid status was determined based on the amount of pituitary TTH and thyroid total triiodothyronine (T3), free thyroxine (T4) hormones. The normal range of hormones was: total T3 - 2.0 - 4.0 pg/ml, free T4 - 8.9 - 17.2 pg/ml, TTH - 0.4 - 4.0 μME/ml, antibodies to thyroperoxidase 0 - 30 mE/ml,
prolactin 66 - 490 mE/ml. l, insulin 4.0 - 23.5 mU/ml.
It was found that the majority of patients with mastopathy (50%) are of late fertile age, and the majority of patients with thyroid pathology (44.5%) are women of early fertile age. (Table 1, Figure 1) It is known that each age period in women is characterised by its own hormonal and metabolic changes.

Table Correlation of age groups with types of mastitis.

	Age groups					
Types of mastitis	18-24 l. of early fertile age		25-34 litres of average fertile age		35-49 litres of late fertile age	
	Abs	%	abs	%	abs	%
Diffuse fibrosis	14	7,61	25	13,59	24	13,04
Cystic form	12	6,52	36	19,57	63	34,24
nodular form	1	0,54	4	2,17	5	2,72
Total	27	14,67	65	35,33	92	50

For this reason, whether it is thyroid disease or MJ disease, each age has its own different form of manifestation (Fig).

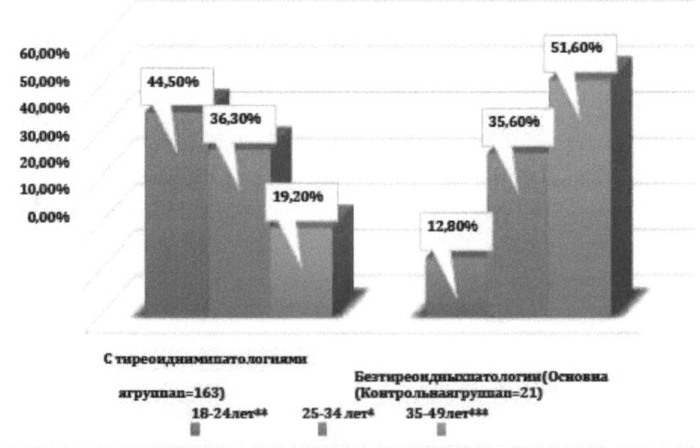

*** $p < 0.001$ - the reliability of the difference between the indicators of both groups is very high.

** p<0.01 - the difference between the indicators of both groups is highly significant.

* p>0.05 - the difference between the indicators of both groups is not significant.

Figure. Prevalence of mastitis among different age groups.

When the patients were categorised by age group, it was found that the main group of patients (44.5%) were women of early fertile (18-24) age, whereas in the control group, women of this age had the least number of patients (12.8%) (p<0.01).

Women of middle fertile age (25-34 years) were observed in almost equal proportions (36.3%/35.6%) between the main group and the comparison group (p>0.05).

Women of late fertile age (35-49 years) made up a significantly smaller proportion (19.2%) of the patients in the main group, while in the control group women of this age were observed the most (51.6%) (p<0.001)

Age classification of patients with various thyroid pathologies. gland.

When dividing patients with various nasal forms of thyroid pathology into age groups, the following situation was revealed (Figure 2). When dividing patients with thyroid pathology by age groups, it was found that the majority of patients with diffuse toxic goitre and thyrotoxic adenoma (66.7%/83.4%, respectively)

women of early childbearing age (18-24 years), while the control group and women of this age were observed the least (12.8%) (p<0.001).

On the contrary, women of late fertile age (35-49 years old) among patients with diffuse toxic goiter and thyrotoxic adenoma were not observed at all, and in the patients who made up the main group, nodular goiter was diagnosed more often (38.2%) than among patients with nodular goiter, and in the control group it was found that women (51.6%) were the most frequently observed (p<0.001).

Risk factors presented in previous studies in women with mastopathy were studied separately (Fig).

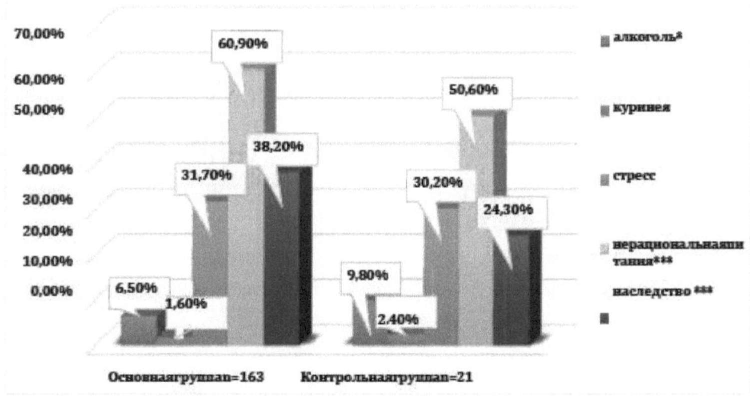

*** p < 0.001 - the reliability of the difference between the indicators of both groups is very high.

** p<0.01 - the difference between the indicators of both groups is highly significant.

Risk factors in patients with mastopathy.

In the examination of patients with bad habits, irrational diet was found in the majority (60.9%/50.6%) of mastopathy patients, followed by acute and chronic stress (61.7%/30.2%), alcohol consumption (6.5%/9.8%), smoking was least observed (1.6%/2.4%).

According to the data on the history of patients with gynaecological risk factors mentioned in the literature and studies conducted before us, the following situation was observed. It was found that 2 or more abortions in the history, primary and secondary infertility were significantly more frequent in the main group of patients compared to the control group ($p < 0.01$). First births at late fertile age were significantly more frequent in the main group of patients than in the control group ($p < 0.001$). The difference between the rates of both groups for information on irregular sexual activity and contraceptive methods was found to be unreliable. ($p>0.05$) According to the anamnestic data collected on the types of contraception included in the risk factors for mastitis, the vast majority (42.4%) of the control group did not use contraception. Intrauterine device (IUD) was the most commonly used contraceptive method (33.33%/35.54% in both groups respectively) and oral contraceptive method was the least commonly used (12%).

The hormonal background of women of reproductive age with mastopathy with thyroid pathology (main group) and without (comparison group) was studied. It was found out that in patients with hypothyroidism of the main group the average level of TTG was 10,59±1,69 μME/ml, 0,299±0,13 μME/ml in patients with hyperthyroidism, 2,34±0,26 μME/ml in patients with euthyroidism, in the comparison group it was 2,27±0,19 μME/ml ($p<0,001$). The mean serum free T4 in hypothyroidism patients in the main group was 9.33±0.77 pg/ml, 19.39±1.33 pg/ml in hyperthyroid patients, 14.75±0.26 pg/ml in euthyroid patients. in the comparison group was 13.89±0.39 pg/ml. was ($p<0.01$). The amount of insulin in serum was 16.77±0.64 mEd/ml in hypothyroid patients and in control group was 13.89±1.94 mEd/l ($p<0.05$). The amount of insulin in serum was 8.5 6±1.12 mE/l in hyperthyroid patients, 9.24±1.12 mE/l in euthyroid patients was not significantly different from the comparison group ($p>0.05$). In comparison At to thyroperoxidase was observed in hypothyroid patients at significantly higher values (284,6 ± 3,36 ME/ml), whereas in hyperthyroid patients it was 186,15 ± 1,12 ME/ml, was ($p<0,05$) 36,4±1,12 ME/ml in euthyroid patients did not differ significantly ($p>0,05$) from the comparison group (28,4±1,12 ME/ml).

Hyperprolactinaemia, which is the main cause of mastitis in most literature, was observed in normal values (296.7 ± 2.23 mIU/l) in patients without thyroid pathology, whereas in hypothyroid patients it was observed in sharply high values (495.6 ± 2.23 mIU/l.) 3.36 IU/ml) ($p<0.05$).

The amount of prolactin in hyperthyroid patients is 238.9± 1.12 IU/ml, was 324.2±1.12 IU/ml in euthyroid patients. ($p<0,05$).

The study investigated the hormonal changes which revealed different forms of mastopathy. Out of 63 patients with diffuse fibrous mastopathy, 34 (53.97 ± 0.86%) had euthyroidism, 23 (36.51 ± 0.44%) had hypothyroidism and 6 (9.52 ± 0.31%) had hyperthyroidism. Hyperprolactinaemia was observed in 20 (31.75 ± 0.29%) of this group and hyperinsulinaemia in 21 (33.33 ± 0.34%). Out of 111 patients with cystic mastopathy in the group, 49 (44.14 ± 0.26%) had hypothyroidism, 48 (43.24 ± 0.24%) had euthyroidism, and 14 (12.61 ± 0.95%) had hyperthyroidism. Hyperprolactinaemia was observed in 33 (29.73 ± 0.83%) of this group and hyperinsulinaemia in 45 (40.54 ± 0.17%).

The association between 3 levels of mastalgia, which is the main clinical sign of mastitis, and the functional state of the thyroid gland was studied. In this case, 72 (39.13±3.60%) of the total number of patients under control had mild pain and 61 (33.15±1.56%) had moderate pain. It was found that 51 patients (24,46±0,97%) had severe, intense pain.

In order to study the influence of thyroid pathology on the clinical course of mastitis, clinical signs of mastitis, mastalgia and lactorrhoea were studied in the main and comparison groups (Fig. 4).

It was found that in the main group of patients mostly (60.9%) non-cyclic mastalgia not related to the menstrual cycle was observed, while in the comparison group this condition was detected in very rare (9.5%) cases ($p<0.001$).

Mastalgia in the main group of patients was predominantly unilateral (62%), whereas in the comparison group this condition was predominantly (57.1%) bilateral ($p<0.01$).

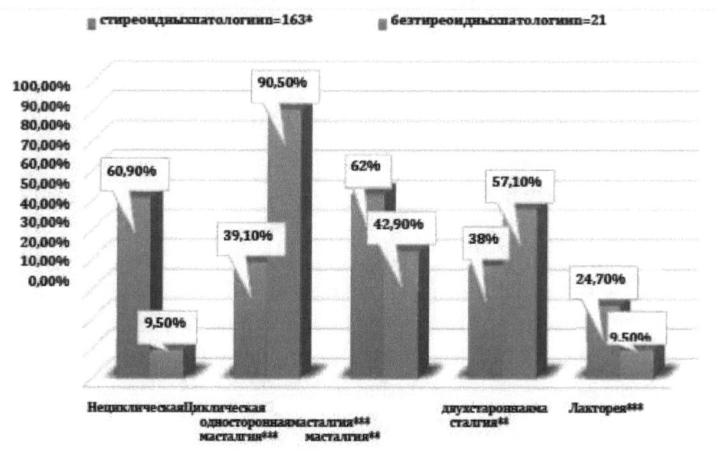

*** $p < 0.001$ - the reliability of the difference between the indicators of both groups is very high.

** $p < 0.01$ - the difference between the indicators of both groups is highly significant.

Influence of thyroid pathology on the clinical course of of mastitis.

In order to study the influence of thyroid pathology on the clinical course of mastitis, we studied the relationship between the 3 levels of mastalgia, the main clinical sign of

mastitis and serum TTG levels (Table 2).
The lowest pain intensity was found in patients with serum TTG levels of 1.0 - 2.0 µIU/ml and 0.4-1.0 µIU/ml, with no significant pain detected in any of the patients.

Relationship between the amount of thyroid hormone and the clinical course of mastitis.

course of mastitis.

№	TSH	Mild pain		Moderate pain		Severe pain		OVERALL	
		abs	%	abs	%	abs	%	abs	%
1	<0,001	7	41,18	8	47,06	2	11,76	17	9,24
2	0,001-0,4	9	69,23	2	15,38	2	15,38	13	7,07
3	0,4-1,0	1	33,33	2	66,67	0	0,00	3	1,63
4	1,0-2,0	20	71,43	8	28,57	0	0,00	28	15,2
5	2,0-3,0	19	70,37	6	22,22	2	7,41	27	14,67
6	3,0-4,0	5	22,73	10	77,27	7	31,82	22	11,96
7	4,0-10	6	15,00	20	50,00	14	35	40	21,74
8	10<	5	14,71	5	14,71	24	70,59	34	18,48
Total		72	39,13	61	33,15	51	24,46	184	100,00

The highest pain intensity scores were noted in patients with subclinical and manifest hypothyroidism (P<0.001).
It was found that most of the patients with mild mastalgia (59.77 ± 1.26 %) were euthyroid patients, while more than half (50.65 ± 1.70 %) of the patients with severe pain syndrome were hypothyroid (p<0.05). No such difference was observed in mastopathy with hyperthyroidism (p>0.05).
In the studies, it was found that patients in the main group had bilateral breast pain unrelated to the menstrual cycle, whereas patients in the comparison group were mainly bothered by pain related to the menstrual cycle and of transient nature.
The BI-RADS study revealed the following breast changes in various thyroid pathologies. In particular, of all the patients (184) included in the study, the majority of them (176/95.6%), showed changes characteristic of BI-RADS categories 1,2,3. When we studied the forms of thyroid pathology in each of these categories, it was found that in the subcategories (BI-RADS 1) a relatively high incidence of nodular goitre in euthyroid state was detected, but as the BI-RADS category increased, their proportion decreased and the proportion of patients with autoimmune thyroiditis increased. In our study BI-RADS 1 is 64 (34.7%) cases of this category. Of these, 26 (14.1%) nodular goitre in euthyroid state, 21 (11.4%) on the background of autoimmune thyroiditis, 4 (2.1%) on the background of diffuse toxic goiter and 1 (0.5%) on the background of thyrotoxic adenoma and 11 of these changes (6%) occurred in the absence of thyroid pathology.
BI-RADS 2 was observed in 38.5% of patients in our study. Of these, 26 (14.1%) were due to nodular goiter, 39 (21.1%) due to autoimmune thyroiditis, 1 (0.5%) due to diffuse toxic goiter and 2 (1%) due to thyrotoxic adenoma.

Clinical and laboratory parameters and ultrasound data of patients identified as BI-RADS type 3 in breast ultrasound findings were followed up for 3 years.
In the study conducted by researchers of Urgench branch of TMA 41 cases of this category. Of these, 12 (29.3%) were due to nodular goiter, 20 (48.8%) to autoimmune thyroiditis, 3 (7.3%) to diffuse toxic goiter and 2 (4.9%) to thyrotoxic adenoma.
All patients were observed in dynamics against the background of treatment every 3-6 months for 3 years. Nineteen patients (10.3%) with reduced or positive changes were included in the BI-RADS -2 category, and 12 (6.5%) patients with negative changes were included in the BI- RADS - 4 category.
In the study, fine needle aspiration biopsy (FNAB) of the breast was performed in 8 patients diagnosed with BI-RADS types 4 and 5 according to breast ultrasound.
In the study conducted by our researchers of Urgench branch of TMA, 6 cases of BI-RADS category - 4 were observed. Of these, 4 (66.8%) were observed in patients with AIT, 1 (16.6%) in patients with DTZ and 1 (16.6%) in patients with thyrotoxic adenoma.
Fine-needle aspiration biopsy was performed in 7 patients diagnosed with BI-RADS 4. As a result, 4 patients were found to have calcified, hypervascular cysts larger than 2-3 cm, and 3 patients were found to have fibroadenomas larger than 5 cm with fibrous cystic mastopathy. All these patients are referred for follow-up to a mammologist. T1N0M0 was detected in the histological report of the only patient in our study who was found to have BIRADS category 5 change. As a result, she underwent unilateral mastectomy and axillary lymphadenectomy and received chemotherapy 5 times.
None of the patients in the study had BI-RADS-6-specific symptoms.
Comparisons of thyroid and breast changes according to the TI-RADS and BI-RADS systems and the effect of treatment of the identified hormonal disorders on mastitis. Comparison of thyroid and mammary glands of the patients included in the study according to the TI-RADS and BI-RADS systems revealed the following (Table).

Interdependence of thyroid and breast changes.

Category on BI RADS	Category no TI-RADS												Total	
	1 n=47		2 n=37		3 n=50		4 n=28		5 n=1		Without thyroid abnormalities, n = 21			
	abs	%	abs	%	abs	%	Abs	%	abs	%	abs	%	abs	%
1 n=59	26	55,32	10	27,03	8	16,00	4	14,29	0	0,00	11	52,38	59	32,07
2 n=77	19	40,43	23	62,16	21	42,00	8	28,57	0	0,00	6	28,57	77	41,85
3 n=40	2	4,26	3	8,11	18	36,00	12	42,86	1	100,00	4	19,05	40	21,74
4 n=6	0	0,00	1	2,70	2	4,00	3	10,71	0	0,00	0	0,00	6	3,26
5 n=1	0	0,00	0	0,00	1	2,00	0	0	0	0,00	0	0,00	2	1,09

total	47	100,00	37	100,00	50	100,00	28	100,00	1	100,00	21	100,00	184	100,00
P	Pearson's chi-square = 58.105; p = 0.001													

In 59 patients with breast changes corresponding to BI-RADS grade I according to ultrasound findings, in (55,32%) patients the changes corresponded to TI-RADS grade I, in 10 of them (27,03%) corresponded to TI-RADS 2, 8 patients (16%) were included in TI-RADS grade 3, in 4 patients (14,29%) the changes included in TI-RADS 4 were determined.

In 77 patients with breast changes corresponding to BI-RADS grade II according to ultrasound findings, 19 (24,6%) patients had changes corresponding to TI-RADS grade I, 23 of them (29,8%) corresponded to TI-RADS grade 2, 21 patients (27,27%) were included in TI-RADS grade 3, 8 patients (10,4%) had changes included in TI-RADS grade 4 and 6 patients had no thyroid pathologies.

In 41 patients with breast changes corresponding to BI-RADS grade III according to ultrasound findings, in 2 (4.9%) patients the changes corresponded to TI-RADS grade I, in 3 (7.3%) corresponded to TI- RADS 2, 19 patients (46.3%) were in TI-RADS grade 3, in 12 patients the changes corresponded to TI-RADS I, in 3 (7.3%) corresponded to TI- RADS 2.

(29.2%) identified changes included in TI-RADS 4, only 1 (2.5%) patient had changes corresponding to TI-RADS 5 and 4 (9.7%) patients had no thyroid pathology. None of the patients in BIRADS 4 degree had thyroid changes according to ultrasound findings corresponding to TI-RADS 1, out of 6 patients 1 (16.7%) corresponded to TI-RADS 2, 2 patients (33.33%) had TI-RADS 3 changes and 3 patients (50%) had TI-RADS 4 changes.

In 1 patient with breast changes corresponding to BI-RADS grade 5, thyroid ultrasound findings showed that these findings corresponded to TI-RADS grade 3.

Patients in BI-RADS group 1,2,3 according to breast ultrasound findings were followed up for 3 years of dynamic follow-up with all the results of clinical and laboratory tests and ultrasound findings, and the efficacy of drug treatment was also monitored. Patients with BI-RADS 4.5 breast changes on ultrasound were subjected to fine needle aspiration biopsy. Based on biopsy results, calcified and hypervascularised cysts measuring 2-3 cm were identified in 3 out of 6 patients. In the remaining 3 patients with cystic fibrosis mastopathy, fibroadenomas larger than 5 cm were identified. The patients were referred for follow-up by a mammological oncologist.

Only 1 patient with BI-RADS 5 underwent mastectomy and histology results revealed $T1N_0M_0$ - transferred under oncologist follow-up.

The degree of mastalgia on the background of treatment of patients with different functional status of the thyroid gland, the conclusion of ultrasound according to BI-RADS system of the breast, the conclusion according to TI-RADS system of the thyroid gland in the pre- and post-treatment period. (Table).

To study the effect of treatment of thyroid pathology on the course of the mastitis.

Thyroid y Status	Degree of mastalgia			BI-RADS categories			THYRADS categories		
	D.L.	P.L.	P	D.L.	P.L.	P	D.L.	P.L.	P
Euthyroidism	4,51±0,17	3,91±0,54	p<0,05	3,45±0,16	3,12±0,21	p>0,05	3,23±0,23	2,94±0,11	p>0,05
Hypothyroidism	7,13±0,36	5,82±0,26	p<0,001	4,87±0,35	3,91±0,55	p<0,001	4,53±0,33	3,66±0,15	p<0,001
Hyperthyroidism 3	4,91±0,85	3,1±0,24	p<0,001	2,85±0,76	2,12±0,71	p<0,05	3,86±0,42	3,12±0,82	p>0,05
Without thyroid Pathologies	4,54±0,36	4,34±0,54	p>0,05	3,56±0,23	3,19±0,04				

D.L. - Before treatment P.L. - After treatment

1 p<0.05 - reliability of differences between main and comparison groups - low

2 * p<0.001 - reliability of differences between main and comparison groups - high

3 ** p<0.01 - reliability of differences between main and comparison groups - mean

Potassium iodide was recommended at a dose of 200 μg/day to patients diagnosed with euthyroid goitre. Numerical pain scale after treatment was from 4.51 ± 0.17 to 3.91 ± 0.54, breast ultrasound score was from 3.45 ± 0.16 to 3.12 ± 0.21 mean BI-RADS, thyroid ultrasound score was reduced from 3.23 ± 0.23 to 2.94 ± 0.11 (p>0.05).

Patients with hypothyroidism and diagnosed mastopathy were recommended levothyroxine sodium at a dose of 1.2-1.6 mcg/kg/day, and the above-mentioned indices were monitored in dynamics. The conclusion of numerical pain scale from 7.13±0.36 to 5.82±0.26 (p<0.001); The conclusion of breast ultrasound decreased in average BI-RADS from 4.87 ± 0.35 to 3.66 ± 0.15 (p<0.001); The conclusion of thyroid ultrasound revealed a decrease in average TI-RADS from 4.53 ± 0.33 to 2.94 ± 0.11 (p<0.001).

Mastopathy patients diagnosed with hyperthyroidism were recommended thiamazole at a dose of 20-30 mg/day, with the above parameters monitored in dynamics. The mastalgia ranged from 4.91 ± 0.85 to 3.1 ± 0.24 (p<0.001); Breast ultrasound findings decreased from an average of 2.85 ± 0.76 to 2.12 ± 0.71 (p<0.05) by BI-RADS; Thyroid ultrasound findings were found to decrease from an average of 3.86 ± 0.42 to 3.12 ± 0.82 (p > 0.05) by TI - RADS.

Many studies have investigated the effect of insulin resistance and hyperinsulinism on the course of mastitis, but since this factor has not been studied in mastitis patients in our region, we focused part of our study on hyperinsulinism and its effect on the course of mastitis (Table).

Correlation between reduction in insulin resistance and clinical signs of mastitis.

	ab	Insulin	Insulin	P	Stepan	Stepan	P	BI	BI	P

	s	DO cure	after treatment		mastalgido treatment	mastalgi and after treatment		RADS categories and up to cure	RADS categorisation and post-treatment	
A	50	19,73±0,14	10,38±0,19	<0,001	5,51±0,27	4,23±0,34	<0,001	3,48±0,12	2,83±0,13	<0,05
B	21	17,43±0,3	16,98±0,3	>0,05	5,35±0,18	5,12±0,46	>0,05	3,43±0,13	3,13±0,83	>0,05

A - treated regularly B - treated irregularly

* p<0.05 - reliability of differences between main and comparison groups - low

2 * p<0.001 - reliability of differences between main and comparison groups - high

3 ** p<0.01 - reliability of differences between main and comparison groups - mean

For this purpose, patients with hyperinsulinism in the study were divided into 2 groups:

A. patients fully compliant with recommendations (diet, physical activity, metformin 1000 mg/day)

B. Patients not complying with the recommendations. Both the dynamics of serum insulin levels and breast ultrasound, BI-RADS report, and the clinical course of mastitis were monitored.

A. Insulin level in the group of patients on the background of treatment was 19.73±0.14 mU/ml. decreased from 10.38±0.19 mU/ml (p<0.001), mastalgia decreased from 5.51±0.27 to 4.23±0.34 (p<0.001), BI-RADS in the conclusion of breast ultrasound decreased from 3.48±0.12 to 2.83±0.13 (p<0.05).

B. In the group of patients the amount of insulin on the background of treatment was 17,43 ± 0,31 mU/ml. decreased from 16,98 ± 0,30 mU/ml (p>0,05), mastalgia decreased from 5,35 ± 0,18 to 5,12 ± 0,46 (p>0,05), and BI-RADS level at ultrasound of mammary glands decreased from 3,43 ± 0,13 to 3,13 ± 0,83 (p>0,05). Thus, treatment of endocrine disorders in patients with mastopathy has a positive effect on the clinical course of the disease and BI-RADS indicators at ultrasound examination (p<0.01).

On the basis of the research "Features of thyroid dysfunctions and mastopathy in women of fertile age of the Southern Priaralie" the following conclusions are made:

1. In women of fertile age in the Southern Priaralie, risk factors for mastopathy are - irrational nutrition (60.9%), acute and chronic stress (61.7%), genetic predisposition (38.2%) of which in (50%) were observed at older fertile age. The presence of thyroid pathology increases the occurrence of mastopathy in early fertile age (44.5%) and in (19.2%) in older fertile age (p<0.001).

2. Thyroid dysfunction is determined in 88.5% of fertile-age women with mastopathy, patients with manifest and severe mastopathy have manifest and subclinical hypothyroidism, implicit mastopathy occurs in those with euteriosis. In patients with plasma TTG level of 1.0 - 2.0 μME/ml, mastopathy is insignificant (71.43±3.54%) in (25.00±3.18%) of patients had moderate pain, also none of the

patients had severe pain. Conversely, patients (70.59±7.81%) with TTG level of 10.0 μME/ml and above had mastitis with severe pain. ($p<0,001$)

3. Treatment of endocrine disorders in patients with mastopathy has a positive effect on the clinical course of disease and on BIRADS ultrasound parameters. In particular, recommendation of levothyroxine sodium 1.2-1.6 μg/kg/day to patients diagnosed with hypothyroidism decreased BI-RADS category from 4.87±0.35 to 3.91±0.15 on average ($p<0.01$); TI-RADS category decreased from 4.53±0.33 to 3.65±0.11 ($p<0.01$), mastalgia decreased from 7.13±0.36 to 5.82±0.26 ($p<0.001$); Recommending metformin 1000 mg daily to patients with insulin resistance decreased mastalgia from 5.51±0.27 to 4.23±0.34 ($p<0.01$), BI-RADS category from 4.1±0.12 to 3, 19±0.13 ($p<0.05$);

4. A correlation was found between TI-RADS category on thyroid ultrasound and BI-RADS category on breast ultrasound in mastopathy patients with thyroid pathology. (Pearson's Chi-square= 58.105; p = 0.001).

5. Treatment of endocrine disorders in patients with mastopathy has a positive effect on the clinical course of the disease and on the BI-RADS system parameters at ultrasound examination. In particular, treatment with thyroid hormones in patients with hypothyroidism led to a decrease in the category of mean BI-RADS from 4.87 to 3.91 ($p<0.01$); TI-RADS category decreased from 4.53 to 3.65 ($p<0.01$), mastalgia decreased from 7.13 to 5.82 ($p<0.001$) reasons; Administration of metformin to patients with insulin resistance reduced mastalgia from 5.51 to 4.23 ($p<0.01$), BI-RADS category on average from 4.1 to 3.19 resulting in a 0.13 ($p<0.05$) reduction.

In the study "Materials and methods of anthropometric examination of the vertebral column in children and adolescents living in the region of the southern Aral Sea region" conducted by researchers of the Urgench branch of the TMA The object of the study were 254 boys, 250 girls permanently residing in the city of Urgench, Khorezm region, 285 boys, 281 girls permanently residing in rural areas of Shavat district. The distribution of children and adolescents by sex, age and place of residence is presented in the table (see Table).

Distribution of the surveyed contingent living in the city according to Groups

	I-group		**II-group**		**111-group**		**IV-rpynna**			
	1-3 years old		Ages 4-7		8-12 years old		13-16 years old		General	
	abs	%	Abs	%	abs	%	abs	%	abs	%
Boys	46	18,1	62	24,4	82	32,3	64	25,2	254	50,4
Girls	48	19,2	55	22,0	80	32,0	67	26,8	250	49,6
Total	94	18,7	117	23,2	162	32,1	131	26,0	504	100

Distribution of the surveyed contingent of rural residents by age periods age periods

	I-group	**II-group**	**111-group**	**IV-rpynna**	
	1-3 years	Ages 4-7	8-12 years old	13-16 years	General

	old						old			
	abs	%	abs	%	Abs	%	abs	%	abs	%
Boys	59	20,7	72	25,3	83	29,1	71	24,9	285	50,4
Girls	72	25,6	77	27,4	74	26,3	58	20,6	281	49,6
Total	131	23,1	149	26,3	157	27,7	129	22,8	566	100

Anthropometric measurements were carried out on the basis of methodological guidelines and methodological recommendations of S.A. Orlov (1997) and N.H. Shomirzaev et al. (1998). For anthropometric measurement of spinal curvatures we have created a useful model "Device for measuring spinal curvatures". Patent No. FAP 02046 dated 08.08.2022 was obtained for the registration of this utility model (see Fig.).

MRI images were used to determine the canal dimensions of the cervical, thoracic, lumbar, and coccygeal spine. The spinal canal in the SI-SVII, TI-TXII, LI-LV, and SI-SIV regions was measured in millimetres (mm).

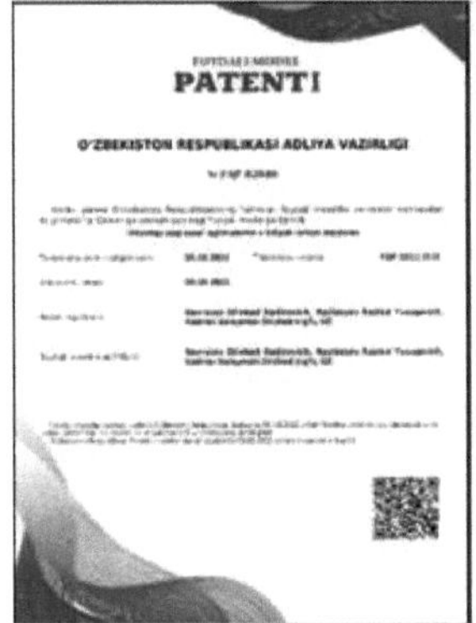

PATENTI

O'ZBEKISTON RESPUBLIKASI ADLIYA VAZIRLIGI

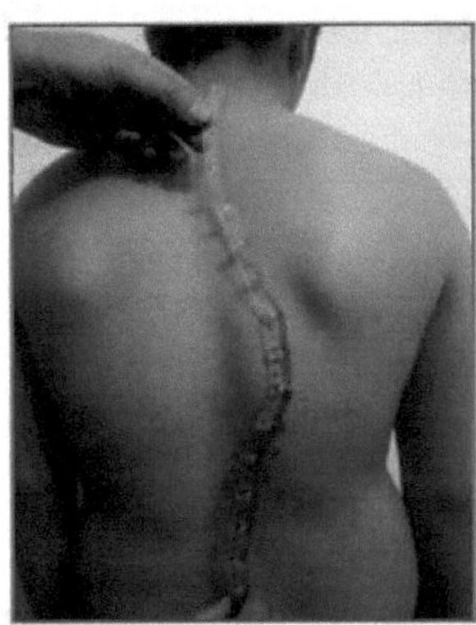

A device for measuring the curvature of the vertebral column

Peculiarities of age-related changes in anthropometric indices of different parts of the spinal column in urban boys 1-16 years old. Measurements of the length of the cervical spine in urban boys show that compared to urban boys 1-3 years old, the length of the cervical spine in boys 4-7 years old ranged from 4.4±0.21 cm to 5.4±0.12 cm (t1=-4.19, increasing to p1<0.0001). In urban boys 8-12 years old, cervical spine length was 6.0±0.61 cm, which was significantly longer than urban boys 1-3 years old. However, compared to previous urban boys 1-3, 4-7 years old, there was a slowing down of cervical spine length growth (t1=-2.362, t2=-0.935, p1=0.020, p2=0.351). In urban boys 13-16 years of age, cervical spine length was 7.1±0.52 cm (t1=-4.167, t2=-2.759, t3=-1.379, p1=0.0001, p2=0.007, p3=0.170).

When measuring the thoracic spine, there was a gradual increase from 15.4±1.23 cm to 31.0±5.63 cm. There was no significant difference in thoracic spine growth in children in the second and third age groups compared to the first age group, and the degree of reliability between the first age group and the adolescent group was high

(t_1=- 2.283, p=0.024).

The lumbar spine, compared to the first age group, in the second and third groups grows in reliable parameters from 5.3±0.16cm to 6.1±0.32cm ($t_{(1)}$=-2.2, $p_{(1)}$<0.030) in 4-8 year old children and to 6.7±0.51cm (t_1=-2.15, t=-2.49, p1=0.034, p_2=0.014), and in the adolescent group it reaches 11.1±0.61cm (t_1=-7.796, $t_{(2)}$=-6.55, t_3=-5.341, p=0.0001, p_2=0.0001, p3=0.0001).

The most reliable growth indicators were obtained when measuring the sacrococcygeal spine. Thus, while in the 1-3 year group this spine section was 4.5±0.14cm, in the second group it reached up to 5.3±0.15cm (t1=-389, p1<0.0001), in the third 6.1±0.34cm (t1=-4.16, t=-2.1, p_1=0.0001, p_2=0.038), and in the adolescent group 10.6±1.23cm (t_1=-4.12, t_2=-3.67, t3=-3.165, p<0.0001, p2=0.0001, p3=0.002).

Measurement of the total length of the spine revealed that at the age of 1- 3 years, the spine length is 29.6±3.4cm. When reaching 4-7 years of age, the spine grows to 36±6.31cm (ti=-0.88, $p_{(1)}$<0.381), in the group of 8-12 years of age, the spine measures 43.7±5.21cm ($t_{(1)}$=-2.21, t=-0.95, $p_{(1)}$<0.029, p_2=0.346), slowing down the growth. As for adolescence, the spine size is 59.8±9.21cm (t1=-2.647, t_2=-1.98, t3=-1.415, p<0.009, p2=0.050, p_3=0.159). This indicates that the change in spine dimensions slows down with age compared to the first group. The increase in spinal column length in boys at the age of 14 years is more intense in the lumbar and thoracic regions compared to the cervical and sacrococcygeal regions.

Peculiarities of age-related changes in anthropometric indices of different parts of the spinal column in rural boys aged 1-16 years. As can be seen in boys living in rural areas there is a reliable growth of the cervical spine in the second and third groups in relation to the first (t_1=-2.04, $p_{(1)}$<0.043, t_1=-3.84, t=-1.74, p_1=0.000, p_2=0.084), and in adolescence there was a significant increase in cervical spine in relation to all previous age groups (t_1=- 6.61, t=-4.38, t=-2.6, p1=0.000 p2=0.000, p3=0.010).

The thoracic spine develops more slowly. While in the 1-3 years group it is 15.1±3.2cm, it reaches 31.61±7.36cm only in adolescence (t1=-1.96, p1=0.052)

Significant differences in the length of the lumbar spine were found between the first group 5.0±0.4 cm, the third group 6.9±0.53 (t_1=- 2.830, $p_{(1)}$=0.005) and especially the adolescent group 11.5±0.56 cm ($t_{(1)}$=-9.19, t=- 7.80, t=- 5.95, p_1=0.0001, p_2=0.0001, p_3=0.0001). The greatest significant differences of all age groups were observed in the growth of the sacrococcygeal spine from 4.3±0.11cm in the first group to 10.9±1.2cm in the fourth group (t_1=-5.11, t=-4.42, t=-3.45, p_1=0.0001, p_2=0.0001, p_3=0.0001). While the total spine length in the group of rural boys 1-3 years old is 28.7±6.23cm, it gradually reaches to 61.15±7.36cm by group 4 (t_1=-3.31, t=-2.2, t=-1.455, p_1=0.001, p_2=0.030, p_3=0.148) per

the cervical, lumbar and sacrococcygeal account.

Age-related changes in anthropometric indices of different parts of the spinal column in urban girls 1-16 years old. In urban girls, compared to the 1-3 years group, the size of the cervical spine increases slightly ($p_{(1)}$<0.509) in the 4-7 years group. In the 8-12 years group, the cervical spine size is significantly larger than the previous groups

(t_1=-4.79, t_2=-2.06, p_1=0.0001, p_2=0.042). However, compared to the previous age, the growth of the cervical spine slowed down to 7.4±0.81cm (ti=-3.08, t2=-2.57, tß=-1.60, pi=0.003, p2=0.011, pz=0.111).

No significant difference was found in the growth of the thoracic spine in children of the second and third age groups compared to the first age group, the degree of reliability between the first age group and the adolescent group is low (t_1=-1.50, $t_{(3)}$=-0.55, p_1=0.136, p3=0.583).

The growth of the lumbar spine, compared to the first group, increases significantly in the 8-12 years group from 5.0±0.15 cm to 6.9±0.82 cm (t_1=- 2.096, p_1=0.038), and reaches 11.3±0.56 cm in the fourth group ($t_{(1)}$=-9.03, t_2=- 7.44, t3=-4.566, p1=0.0001, p2=0.000, p3=0.0001).

When measuring the sacrococcygeal spine, it was found that while in the 1-3 year group this spine was 4.3±0.4cm, in the second group it reached up to 5.6±0.11cm (t_1=-3.28, $p_{(1)}$<0.001), but in the third group there was a slowing down of growth compared to the second group 6.5±0.61cm (t_1=-2.893, t_2=-1.407, p_1=0.005 p_2=0.162). The fourth group showed a significant increase with respect to all previous groups 10.9± 1.24cm (t1=-4.24, t2=-3.67, t3=-2.95, p1=0.0001, p_2=0.0001, p3=0.004).

The total length of the spine gradually increases from 28.6±5.83 cm in the first group to 60.7±12.4 cm in the fourth group (t_1=-2.02, p_1=0.046). The increase in the length of the vertebral column in girls aged 13-16 years in the cervical and sacro- coccygeal regions is more intense compared to the thoracic and lumbar regions.

Age-related changes in anthropometric indicators of different parts of the spinal column in rural girls aged 1-16 years. According to the data, as in urban girls, the cervical spine of rural girls in the second group increases slightly ($p_{(1)}$<0.588) compared to the first age group. In the third age group, cervical spine size is significantly larger than previous groups 5.9±0.43 cm (t1=- 2.31, $t_{(2)}$=-2.12, p1=0.023, p_2=0.035). In adolescence, the length of the cervical spine is 7.36±0.12 cm. (t1=- 6.03, t_2=-6.58, t_3=-3.25, p1=0.000, p_2=0.000, p_3=0.001), slowing down compared to c 8-12 years.

The thoracic spine develops slowly, no significant numerical differences were observed in each age group, although the length of the thoracic spine was significantly longer from 14.8±3.75 cm to 30.9±8.12 cm compared to the first group.

The lumbar spine of rural girls starts to grow intensively in the group of 8-12 years of age compared to the first years of life. Especially the growth of the lumbar spine increases significantly during adolescence, reaching 11.1±1.02 cm (ti=-4.60, t_2=-4.449, t3=-3.969, pi=0.0001, p_2=0.0001, p_3=0.0001). The sacrococcygeal region is also formed from 4.1±0.81 cm to 10.7±0.91 cm (ti= -5.03, t2=-5.15, t3=-4.59, pi=0.0001, p2=0.0001, p3=0.0001).

The total length of the spine in the first age group is 28±6.36 cm, only by adolescence it reaches 60.3±12.3 cm at the expense of the lumbar and sacrococcygeal sections. In the second and third age groups, the growth of the spinal column slows down, and by the period of puberty, 13-16 years of age, a new acceleration of its growth is observed.

Growth and body mass indices in children 1-16 years old living in rural and urban areas. The development of the spine and its compartments correlates with the physical development of the organism, especially body weight and height. Differences in height were found between urban and rural boys and girls. While the height of urban boys 1-3 years of age was 85.9±3.2 cm, rural boys 80.8±4.56 cm, urban girls 84.2±0.43 cm, rural girls had a length of 80.6±7.21 cm. In adolescence, rural boys grow more than their urban counterparts, 159.7±6.3 cm compared to 163.9±7.3 cm. The height of urban and rural girls remains about the same. There is no statistically significant difference in height between urban and rural children, but a trend of difference was found. Both urban boys and girls of the first three years of life weigh (13.6±2.36kg and 13.5±3.12kg) slightly more than rural boys (12.8±2.31kg and 12.3±1.91kg). However, from the age of four years onwards, these figures flatten out somewhat. By adolescence, rural boys (57.3±8.54kg) weigh more than urban boys (54.9±13.3kg), but urban adolescent girls weigh more than rural girls (52.4±12.6kg and 48.9±6.65kg).

"Comparative characteristics of age, sex and regional changes in anthropometric parameters of the spinal column of children 1-16 years old" describes the results of the study of the dynamics of changes in anthropometric parameters of the spine, body weight and height in children and adolescents 1-16 years old living in urban and rural areas, a comparative analysis was carried out.

Comparative analysis of anthropometric parameters of the cervical spinal column in children 1-16 years old living in urban and rural areas. As can be seen from the diagram data, in boys and girls 1-3 years of age, the cervical spine averaged 15% of the total length of the entire vertebral column, and by adolescence it was up to 11.8%. The length of the cervical spine increased 1.7 times compared to 1-3 year olds, 1.24 times compared to 4-7 year olds and 1.18 times compared to 8-12 year olds.

Body weight, height and total spine length in urban children aged 1-16 years. aged 1-16 years.

	Age categories	Height (cm)	Weight (kg)	Length of the vertebral column (cm)
I-group	1-3 years old	88,1±3,2	13,5±2,36	29,1±3,4
11-group	Ages 4-7	112,9±4,29	19,7±4,3	35,7±6,31
Ill-group	8-12 years old	136.3±11,1	34,7±6,3	43,7±5,1
group IV	13-16 years old	159,6±6,3	53,6±6,2	60,2±6,21

Body weight, height and total spine length. of rural children aged 1-16 years.

	Age categories	Height (cm)	Weight (kg)	Length of the vertebral column (cm)
I-group	1-3 years old	80,7±4,56	12,5±2,31	28,3±3,27
II- group	Ages 4-7	110,4±8,71	20,4±4,65	34,8±5,5
III- group	8-12 years old	137,3±11,2	33,4±6,31	44,2±4,3
IV- group	13-16 years	160,9±6,3	53,1±8,54	60,7±5,1

	old			

Thus, based on the data obtained and presented above during the anthropometric study, boys and girls 1-3 and 4-7 years old (I and Il-group) living in the city have an advantage in anthropometric indicators of the vertebral column compared to their peers living in rural areas. Boys 8-12 and 13-16 years old (Group III and IV) living in rural conditions have an advantage in the dynamics of growth of the vertebral column compared to their peers living in the city. The dynamics of changes in anthropometric indicators of the vertebral column in boys and girls 1-16 years old is associated with the influence of the environment (rural and urban areas), sex, age and physical development indicators (body weight and height).

According to the results of the research "Age peculiarities of anthropometric indices of different parts of the vertebral column in children up to adolescence living in the Southern Aral Sea region" the following conclusions are made:

1. There was no statistically significant difference between the absolute values of total spine length in boys living in urban and rural areas in different age groups, while the absolute values of total spine length up to the age of 7 years were predominant in urban children, and from the age of 8 years became dominant in children living in rural areas.

This condition manifested itself in all parts of the spine and especially in the cervical spine.

2. The absolute values of the total length of the spine of urban and rural girls in different age groups were almost the same. The absolute length of the lumbar and sacrococcygeal spine was greater in urban girls than in rural girls.
3. While the growth of urban children in the 1-3 year age group was 13.6 per cent greater than that of rural children, this difference decreased sharply in the next age group (more than 2.9 per cent in the 4-7 year age group), became almost equal in the 8-12 year age group, and from 13-16 years onwards it became dominant among rural children. This condition was manifested in all spine regions and especially in the cervical spine. Body weight in urban and rural children in different age groups did not differ practically until adolescence, when in adolescence (13-16 years) body weight in rural children began to prevail over that of urban children.
4. Changes in the growth of urban and rural boys at different age groups reversed the trend for children in the general group and from 8-12 years of age, the superiority of rural children became evident. While body weight of urban and rural boys is about the same at 1-3 and 4-7 years of age, at age 812, the weight of urban boys begins to dominate rural boys, and in adolescence (13-16 years), on the contrary, the weight of rural boys began to dominate that of their urban counterparts.
5. The height of urban girls in the 1-3 years age group was 12.7 per cent higher than that of rural girls, while in the following age groups there was virtually no difference in the height of the two groups of girls compared. Body weight of urban and rural girls, as well as body length, did not differ until adolescence. During adolescence (13-

16 years of age), the weight of rural girls began to dominate that of urban girls.

Diagram on the impact on the organism of environmental factors in the region Southern Priaralie (by R.B.Abdullaev. and A.M.Bakhtiyarova)

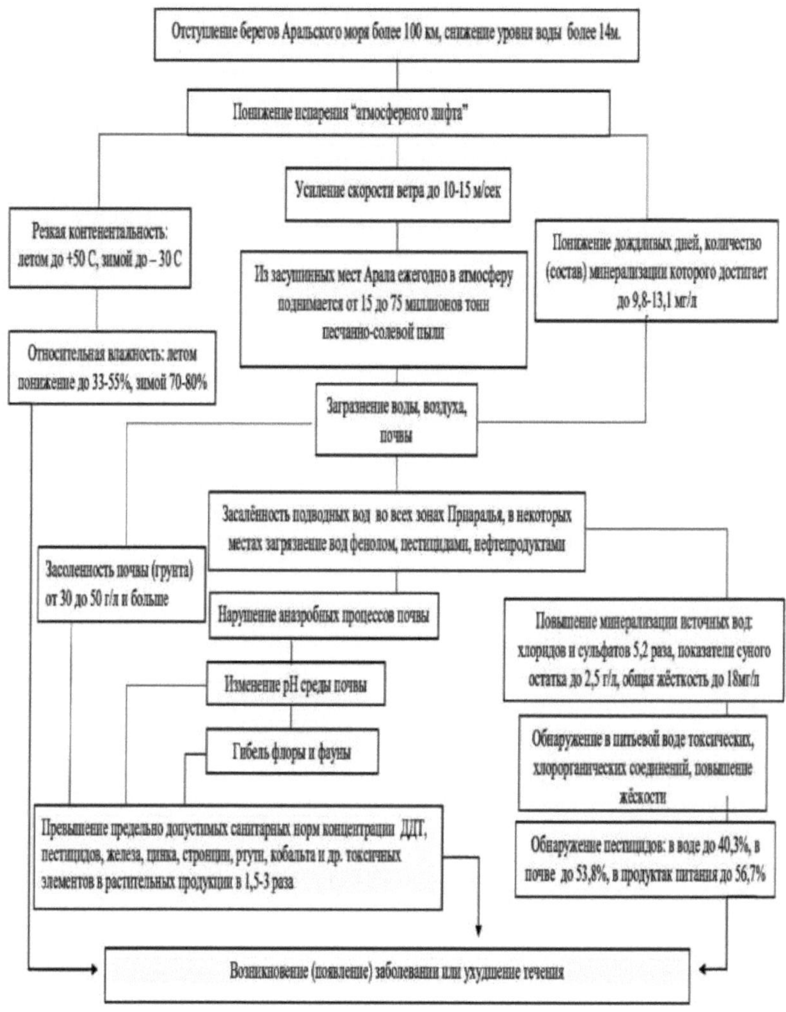

According to MHI String water quality control by Khorezm SIAC for the 4th quarter of 2022.

№	Selection site (facility)		IIIIIII	Discharge point	Wastewater discharge thousand m3/day	Date of selection	Iigerediepts content, mg/d.m3														
							Sample cohort pcs	pH	paci kne-d	BOD5	Platoon. milestone	Dry residue	CI.	SO4	NO2	N114	NO3	Fe	P	Cg+6	Zn
									mgO_2/dm'	mgOUdm'.	mg/dm^3	mg/dm^3	mg/dm^3	mg/dm^3	mg/dm^3	mg/dm^3	mg/dm"	mg/dm^3	mg/dm^3	mg/dm^3	mg/dm^3
1	2	3	4	5	6	7	8	9	10	11	12	13	14	15	16	17	18	19	20	21	22
1	"GURLAN. GLOBAL TEKS." MCHJ	receipts	307480031	Shanti kall-tor	700	18.10.2022	1	8.77	off	75	199	2100	819	915	1.6	10	5	4.6	0,64	0,206	0.172
		reset					1	8.3	off	40	60	1794	663	720	2,34	1.4	3.4	0,54	0.09	0,056	0,54
		above					1	7.79	9.2	13,5	141	1356	234	280	0,64	3.2	1,2	0,38	0,264	0,054	0.496
		below					1	8.4	7,7	20	79	1554	351	410	0,46	5	1.6	0,96	0,02	0,12	0,728
2	"Uztex Group" MSCH	receipts	204651661		28	14.12.2022	1	7,42	OTS	45	520	2850	670	740	6,4	11,2	3.75	1,16	0,8	0,08	1,34
		reset					1	7,39	0,6	37,5	384	2390	574	620	1,76	10,4	3,4	0,5	0,72	0,056	1,008
		above					1	7,62	6,2	17	165	1780	415	465	0,86	8,8	1	0,4	0,496	off	0,472
		below					1	7,5	0,78	20	272	2150	510	550	1,04	10	2	0,48	0,6	0,03	0,728
3	"KHOREZM TECH" .mj	concrete No. 1	302413758		25	27.10.2022	1	9	off	69	210	1935	479	500	0,2	12,8	6	0,16	0,64	0,26	0,892
		concrete No. 2					1	9.3	OTS	75	235	1990	574	540	0,24	14	7.8	0,18	0,76	0,294	0,96
4	"Hazorasp textil" by MZH	CNS	300074865			14.11.2022	1	7.54	off	37,5	165	1189	287	350	5,82	11,2	5	1,54	0,264	0,254	0,12
5	"TEXTILE FINANCE KHOREZM" MJ	receipts	304758460	R. Poliazov kall-tor	46,8	03.11.2022	1	7,87	0,3	25	87	2300	606	700	6,4	12	5.4	1,82	0,17	0,23	0,54
		reset					1	7,57	0,78	15	52	1935	467	560	5,44	8	3.4	0,64	OD	0,05	0,4
		above					1	7,7	1,57	7,5	29	2460	510	706	5,6	3,4	5	0,25	0,002	OTS	0,356
		below					1	7,71	1,6	10	42	2180	479	654	5,78	5,4	4,8	0,36	0,008	0,01	0,38
6	Urgench O.C	receipts	201733481	Chakkakul call-tor	81	08.11.2022	1	9.6	ague	100	305	2320	670	705	2,48	13,6	8.8	2,88	0,64	0,3	0,96
		reset					1	9.05	off	95	195	2140	638	660	1,76	11.2	7,2	2.24	0,56	0,26	0,82
		above					1	7,55	6,9	20	PO	1350	415	440	0,6	3	1.6	0,1	0,14	0,0032	0.076
		below					1	8,15	5,3	21.2	155	1480	467	510	0,86	5.4	2.4	0.76	0,168	0,11	0,188
7	Yupnak O.C	receipts	201733481	Chikirchikal l-tor	11	08.11.2022	1	8,92	OTS	55	260	1520	467	495	0,64	13,6	3.4	0.8	0,76	0,4	0,704
		reset					1	8,65	4	40	175	1410	415	460	0,46	11,2	2.9	0,48	0,56	0,096	0,66
		above					1	7,24	7,5	13,7	75	1100	319	365	0,32	2,6	1	0.16	0,324	OTS	0,096
		NIJS					1	7,4	7,1	20	95	1240	383	405	0,34	5,4	1.2	0,28	0,4	0,0432	0.356

8	HivaO.S.	iiocryimuw	201733481	Ozörpykal l-tor	10	08.11.2022	1	9,05	ore	79	230	1660	510	540	0.8	12	3,75	2,04	0,68	0,188	0,796
		reset					1	8,94	off	65	160	1520	467	500	0,64	10	2,4	1,6	0,56	0,126	0,68
		above					1	7,62	7,1	17,5	105	1290	319	375	0,86	2,8	2,9	0,64	0,22	0,0098	0,12
		below					1	8,05	6,5	22	125	1410	351	415	1,28	5	3,75	0,8	0,3	0,021	0,16
9	MFJ shaklndagi "Hina" chet el korhonasi	receipts	200427499		90	21.11.2022	1	8,12	4,75	30	85	1150	319	340	0,14	4,6	2,2	0,36	0,308	0,0098	0,588
		reset					1	8,35	5.3	20	65	996	287	302	0,5	4.2	3,6	0.26	0,3	0,0096	0,564
		above					1	7,48	7,4	10	95	1310	351	375	0,24	2	2,7	0,16	0,28	0,0092	0,496
		below					1	8	7,07	13,5	105	1240	319	350	0,2	2,4	2,4	0,2	0,288	0,0094	0,54
10	"HonkaDon mahsulotlari" AJ	receipts	200429242	Mityanov call-tor	80	28.11.2022	1	8,58	off	35	55	1560	351	405	1,44	6,4	8,8	0,54	0,8	0,224	1,244
		reset					1	8,42	arc	25	30	1370	287	365	128	2,4	7.8	0,48	0,624	0,054	0,844
		above					1	8,05	off	2,5	45	860	128	180	1,36	2.8	1.8	0,1	0,018	0,0002	0,54
		below					1	8,18	4	3,75	35	920	191	250	1.2	2,6	22	0,16	0,042	0,005	0,598
11	"Korakoshtaymir Plastic Service x'k	reset	205334169	Zhirmnzkul kall-tor	50-70	20.12.2022	1	7,59	off		126	1540	383	420	0,74	3	2,7	0,46	0,8	0,056	1,372
		above					1	7,31	2,1		118	1410	319	360	0,6	2,8	1.2	0,02	0,012	0,0092	0,94
		below					1	7,45	off		278	1650	351	390	0,7	2,6	2	0,38	0,3	0,019	1,152

Statistical data 2022-2023 according to the Department of Ecology and Environmental Protection of Khorezm province

By MIZ Kosh role of string water quality by Khorezm SIAC for the 4th quarter of 2023.

№	Selection site (object)		TIN	Discharge point	Wastewater discharge thousand m3/day	Date of selection	Contents of the nnge [ESD11C1HGOV, mg/dmS														
							Number of samples pcs	pH	plant kiss-d	BOD5	Platoon. thing	Dry residue	CL	SO4	NO2	NII4	NO3	Fe	P	Cg+6	Zn
									m|O d 'dm	mgO₂/dm	mg/dm3	mg/dm³	mg/dm³	mg/dm³	mg/dm³	mg/dm³	mg/dm³	mg/dm³	mg/dm³	mg/dm³	mg/dm³
1	2	3	4	5	6	7	8	9	10	11	12	13	14	15	16	17	18	19	20	21	22
1	"GURLAN . GLOBAL TEKS." MSCH	receipts	307480031	Shanti kall-tor	700	05.12.2023	1	7	ore	14	40	1520	351	390	0,135	off	0,121	0,06	0,36	0,0132	0,026
		reset					1	7,08	orc	10	32	1206	287	325	0,114	off	0,104	0,04	0,32	0,01	0,022
		above					1	7,4	U	5,75	23	1008	223	260	0,03	off	0,016	0,03	off	off	off
		below					1	7,35	1,1	8,25	27	1100	255	265	0,045	off	0,022	0,02	0,06	off	off
2	"KHOREZM TECH" BFM	concrete No. 1	302413758		25	21.11.2023	1	7,9	off	22,5	84	1480	319	370	0,225	1,232	0,638	0,74	0,19	0,108	0,08
		concrete No. 2					1	7,65	off	28,7	63	1220	287	330	0,18	1,155	0,616	0,66	0,11	0,084	0,076
3	"Hazorasp textil" by MZH	KIS	300074865			26.10.2023	1	7,55	off	37,5	83	1474	383	440	0,519	6,779	0,572	0,38	0,44	0,0036	0,09
4	Urgench O.S.	receipts	201733481	Chakkakul call-tor	81	28.11.2023	1	8,3	off	75	95	2170	447	510	0,93	5,39	1,045	1,2	0,6	0,116	0,608
		reset					1	7,8	ore	65	80	1860	415	470	0,84	5,082	0,869	0,9	0,52	0,092	0,58
		above					1	7	1,1	8,5	28	1120	255	290	0,234	0,85	0,286	0,25	0,2	off	0,148
		below					1	7,2	1	12,5	37	1270	319	370	0,3	1,078	0,308	0,3	0,26	0,0028	0,17
5	Pitnak O.S.	receipts	201733481	Chikirchikal l-tor	11	28.11.2023	1	7,95	0,5	45	70	1650	383	**420**	0,69	3,85	0,726	0,68	0,46	0,064	0,08
		reset					1	7,73	0,8	38	48	1356	350	400	0,552	3,388	0,682	0,56	0,38	0,038	0,056
		above					1	7,25	1,7	5,5	20	1150	223	270	0,135	0,77	0,132	0,25	0,14	off	off
		below					1	7,45	1,5	7,5	33	1200	255	310	0,165	0,924	0,154	0,28	0,19	off	off
6	Hiva O.S.	receipts	201733481	Ozeriikal l-tor	10	28.11.2023	1	8,15	off	65	80	1700	383	450	0,78	4,312	0,869	0,78	0,52	0,084	0,58
		reset					1	8	off	55	68	1580	319	400	0,639	3,542	0,726	0,66	0,44	0,06	0,512
		above					1	7.5	1,3	7,5	25	1060	223	270	0.195	0,73	0,203	0,32	0,184	off	0,096
		below					1	7,85	1Д	8,5	40	1100	255	310	0,234	0,85	0,253	0,38	0,24	off	0,102
7	"Korakosh Ta'mir Plastic Service" x/k	reset	205334169	Jirmizkul kall-tor	50-70	08.11.2023	1	7,35	off	32,5	65	1618	319	360	0,18	0,077	0,049	0,1	0,44	0.0028	0,026
		above					1	7,41	1,6	3,75	40	1390	255	300	0,015	тос	0,0055	off	0,04	off	off
		below					1	7,45	1,8	5,75	45	1436	287	330	0,03	off	0,011	off	0,05	off	off
8	"Feedgran" MSH	concrete/chukur	301316238			23.11.2023	1	7,56	1,19	15	25	1078	255	300	0,075	ore	off	0,01	off	off	off
9	"OASIS S DREAM" MSH	reset	306412717			06.12.2023	1	7,88	1,1	13	58	1080	255	305	off	off	off	0,02	0,04	0,032	0,026
		above					1	7,51	1,6	5	66	1468	351	390	off	off	off	0,03	0,1	0,01	0,038
		below					1	7,7	1,3	7,5	60	1400	319	360	off	off	off	off	0,03	0,01	off

Khorezm Oblast Monitoring Department Report for 2023. **/Atmosphere/.**

Srsd.quarter.

№	Name of the company	Names and roles of S1va, workshop, section	The following are examples of technologies, equipment, etc.	Controlled source number		Nanmeno-bath of the ingredient to be determined	Project, concentrations mg/mS	Design emission value (according to the normative document), g/sec	Actual concentrations mg/mS	Actual Emissions /sec.	II rivers incline and norm at ive (MAP, DH) how many pai	Presence and type of dust-legal unit (DGO)	WU purification efficiency, %		Measures taken			Number of controllable sources.
				blueprint	fact								Project.	fact.	CoAO Ruth article number	on.too.ine sum ipraf 114 C. sum	write-in of shares amount of penalty ths.soum	
1	2	3	4	5	6	7	8	9	10	11	12	13	14	15	16	17	18	**19**
1	**"Urgench yog moi" AJ Urganch city**	Milling shop	Aspirate.	78	78	Dust.meal	98,1	0,127	85,933	0,112	-	4BCSH	**90**	90				2
				79	79	Dust.meal	113,76	0,1317	103,099	0,127	-	UTS-38-500	**88,4**	88				
2	"Khoratm shakar" MCHJ. Tuprakkalja r/n	Boiler house	Boilers of the brand "RAKET SHG 2 CHT	17	17	Nitrogen dioxide	82,95	1,43	81,503	0,872	-	-	-	-	-	-	-	14
						Carbon oxide	364,72	6.37	275	2,941								
				18	18	Nitrogen dioxide	82.95	1,43	79,508	0,85	-		-	-	-	-	-	
						Carbon oxide	364,72	6,37	262,5	2,807								
3	"WBM Qoshkopir clastc-GMJ".	Drying compartment.	Sep-CC-15	2	2	Dust slam.	35	0,073	30,39	0,064	-	CS6-.	96	96				**4**
				9	9	Dust slam.	43,749	0,091	42,476	0,085	-	CS6-1200	98	96				
4	"Khorazmteh" MJ Clastesri.	Drying compartment.	Sep-CC-15	5	5	CHLOE Dust.	38,1	0,073	36,471	0,072	-	CS6-.	90	89			Raz ra. nov	6
				6	6	Dust slam.	52,5	0,109	45,445	0,095	-	CS6-1200	90	90			pdw	
			Aspiration system	7	7	Dust slam.	43,75	0,091	33,105	0,086		CS6-1200	90	90				
5	TEXTILE FINANCE KHOREZM 2 catheg-e Shawat pahta toz.	Drying compartment.	Sep-CC-15	3	3	Dust slam.	62,749	0,157	54,027	0,136		CS 6-CS	90	89				4
				4	4	Dust slam.	67,335	0,157	59,862	0,149		CS6-.	90	90				
		Heads, cor	**Aspiration system**	6	6	Dust slam.	52,5	0,109	43,19	0,104		CS6-.	90	90				
				8	8	Dust slam.	43,749	0,091	31,344	0,066		CS6-1200	93	93				
6	"Urganch bahmal." BFM	Boiler house	turkish cateel ESB-1000.1pc	5	5	Nitrogen dioxide	57,973	0,32216	59,383	0,21		-	-	-				4
						Carbon oxide	126,54	0,4274	75	0,266		-	-	-				
7	"URGENCH CLUSTER " BFM	SOC.OC	Sep-CC-15	4	4	Dust slam.	68,235	0,1575	57,528	0,141		CS6-.	90	90				4
				5	5	Dust slam.	38,1	0.0731	24,685	0,062		CS 6-VZP1200	96	96				
8	"Gurlan Global Tex" MZH (Gurlen r/n) 2 catheg-e	**social. ots** Main, corpus.	SS-15.	1	1	Dust slam.	-	-	26,4	0,11		CS6-.	90	89				9
			Press.lint.	2	2	Dust slam.	-	-	27,578	0,11		Csb-	90	89				
			asperation	3	3	Dust slam.	-	-	38,85	0,125		CS6-.	90	90				
9	"Yangi Ariq Teh" MSJ (Yangiarik district) 2 catheg-e	SOC. ots Main building.	SS-15.	3	3	Dust slam.	62,749	0,157	39,323	0,114		Ц8-	90	9				3
				6	6	Dust slam.	52,5	0,109	32,93	0,079		Ц8-	90	89				
				8	8	Dust slam.	43,749	0,091	40,993	0,082		Ц8-	90	90				
10	-KOBOTEX-MCJ Bogatsky district	SOC. ots Main, corpus.	SS-15.	*3*	3	Dust slam.	62,749	0,157	63,072	0,144		CS6-.	90	89				3
			Press.lint.	6	6	Dust slam.	52.5	0,109	41,791	0,088		CS6-.	90	89				
			asperation	8	8	Dust slam.	43,749	0,091	42,081	0,089		CS 6-VZP	90	90				
11	"Bohodirhon Egam. coals "X/K. 2-category.	Colz.pec. Kiln brick	Pipe	9	9	Nitrogen dioxide	17,096	0,095	15,912	0,087		-						4
						Carbon oxide	82,239	0,457	65	0,358		-						
12	"Allabergan ota." CHTHF. 2-category.	Colz.pec. Kiln brick	Pipe	II	11	Nitrogen dioxide	-	-	14,387	0,079		-						3
						Carbon oxide	-	-	25	0,137		-						
13	Zhaikhun yu/tardan muntaeam foidolanish" CC. Urganç t	Asphalt shop	Cyc.fyltr	1	1	Nsorgai.dust			-	-	-	-						-
									-	-	-	-						

№	Name	Source	Type			Substance												
14	"Mahmoud" MJW Urgench, r/n 2-cat.	Colz.pec. Kiln brick	Pipe	9	9	Nitrogen dioxide	22,164	0.068	18,97	0,058		-						3
						Carbon oxide	170,367	0,524	137,5	0,423		-						
15	"NAWRUZ" MJ Urgench, r/n 2-cat.	Colz.pec. Kiln brick	Pipe	11	11	Nitrogen dioxide	27,297	0,151	25,172	0,091		-						1
						Carbon oxide	36,213	0,201	35,75	0,158		-						
16	Boburbek Rustam Yusuf MSJ Gurlant 2-cat	Colz.pec. Kiln brick	Pipe	1	1	Nitrogen dioxide	-	-	-	-								-
						Carbon oxide	-	-	-	-								
17	"Amin Buron Mirzo" PE Yangibazar.r/n 2-cat.	Colz.pec. Kiln brick	Pipe	1	1	Nitrogen dioxide	-	-	14,544	0,033		-						2
						Carbon oxide	-	-	70	0,161		-						
18	"ALLABERGAN "HICHF Yangibazar.r/n 2-cat.	Colz.pec. Kiln brick	Pipe	10	10	Nitrogen dioxide	17,059	0,061	10,895	0,038		-						4
						Carbon oxide	46,991	0,172	28,8	0,101		-						
19	"MADIR" PE Hankinsky.r/n 2-cat.	Colz.pec. Kiln brick	Pipe	10	10	Nitrogen dioxide	37,97	0,211	18,083	0,1		-						3
						Carbon oxide	125,97	0,7	70	0,388		-						
20	"Zhaikhun Kurilish" MZH Hankinsky.r/n 2-cat.	Colz.pec. Kiln brick	Pipe	11	11	Nitrogen dioxide	14,654	0,074	13,046	0,072		-						3
						Carbon oxide	86,55	0,459	57,5	0,319		-						
21	"Badrhonli Pirhon" HC Khivin. r/n 2-cate.	Colz.pec. Kiln brick	Pipe	11	11	Nitrogen dioxide	23,5	0,132	13,489	0,074		-						3
						Carbon oxide	26,4	0.141	20	0,11								
22	"Kuchtsor bogbon" HC. Khivin. r/n 2-cate.	Colz.pec. Kiln brick	Pipe	1	1	Nitrogen dioxide	-	-	13,043	0,069		-						4
						Carbon oxide			41,25	0,218								
23	"Otonazar "fx Khivin. r/n 2-cate.	Colz.pec. Kiln brick	Pipe	9	9	Nitrogen dioxide	27,297	0,083	13,476	0,047								3
						Carbon oxide	36,123	0,638	137,5	0,481								
24	"Khiva Ahmad usta" HC Khivin. r/n 2-cate.	Colz.pec. Kiln brick	Pipe	II	11	Nitrogen dioxide		0,088	19,353	0,06								3
						Carbon oxide		0,112	32.5	0,101								
25	"Khiva Fays HC Khivin. r/n 2-cate.	Colz.pec. Kiln brick	Pipe	1	1	Nitrogen dioxide		0,113	14,882	0,082								3
						Carbon oxide		0,155	20	0,11								
26	"Bunyodbek Ergashbek." Yangibazar. r/n 2-cate.	Colz.pec. Kiln brick	Pipe	1	1	Nitrogen dioxide	-	-	-	-								-
						Carbon oxide	-	-	-	-								
27	Shohrukh tadbirkor HC Honka. r/n 2-cate.	Colz.pec. Kiln brick	Pipe	11	11	Nitrogen dioxide	9,537	0,053	7,46	0,041								3
						Carbon oxide	59,565	0,331	45	0,247								
28	"Hazarasptexsteel." MCH 2-cat	socio	SS-15.	3	3	Fervour CHLOP	62,749	0,157	60,407	0,151								4
			asperation	6	6	Dust HLOP.	52,5	0,109	26,093	0,076								
29	Khiva Cluster" MCH Hiwat2-cat	social	SS-15.	1	1	Dust HLOP.	-	-	16,788	0,203								5
		Head cor	asperation	2	2	Dust HLOP.	-	-	22,112	0,267								
30	UzAvto Motors" AZh Khorezm phil. 1-cate.	Wearable	Pipe	1	1	Nitrogen dioxide	40,2	0,0317	26,706	0,022								7
						Carbon oxide	128,5	0,105	90	0,075								
31	GREAT COTTON EXPORT MJW. Rich t. 2 cat.	sococ	SS-15.	1	1	Dust HLOP.	-		63,147	0,157								2
		Chief. to		2	2	Dust HLOP.	-		58,624	0,123								
32	' Xudaybergan Abdol" HC Organdi t. 2-category.	Colz.pec. Kiln brick	Pipe	9	9	Nitrogen dioxide	-		8,254	0,045								1
						Carbon oxide	-		25	0,137								
33	'Norimon Xoji' Urganch T. 2-category.	Colz.pec. Kiln brick	Pipe	1	1	Nitrogen dioxide	-		14,27	0,049								1
						Carbon oxide	*		37,5	0,131								
34	"Goibugishtta'aminot "hk Urgench t. 2-category.	Colz.pec. Kiln brick	Pipe	10	10	Nitrogen dioxide	23,38	0,13	21,328	0,117								4
						Carbon oxide	183,01	1,017	100	0,55								
35	'Anjirchi g'isht' MChJ	Colz.pec. Kiln brick	Pipe	1	1	Nitrogen	-	-	10,62	0,037								1

	Urganch t. 2-categ.					dioxide												
						Carbon oxide	-	-	20	0,07								
36	Izzat Komil XK Bog'ot T. 2-category.	Colz.pec. Kiln brick	Pipe	1	1	Nitrogen dioxide			7,593	0,04								2
						Carbon oxide			32,5	0,172								
37	"Shovot Abror g'isht qurilish" xk Shovot t, 2-category	Colz.pec. Kiln brick	Pipe	1	1	Nitrogen dioxide	-	-	10,73	0,041								1
						Carbon oxide	-	-	28,75	0,109								
38	"Shoxobod qurilish servis' Shovot t, 2-category	Colz.pec. Kiln brick	Pipe	1	1	Nitrogen dioxide	-	■	11,263	0,043								1
						Carbon oxide	-	-	25	0,095								
39	"Boyot g'isht" XK Yangiariq t. 2-category.	Colz.pec. Kiln brick	Pipe	10	10	Nitrogen dioxide	26,938	0,149	38,315	0,13								1
						Carbon oxide	206,874	1,149	100	0,34								
40	"Yangibazar agro cluster" мсн. Yangibazart. 2 cat.	soc.oc	SS-15.			Dust HLOP.	-	-	-	-								-
		Chief. to				Dust HLOP.	*	-	-	-								
																		125

Statistical data 2022-2023 according to the data of the Department of Health Care of Khorezm province

Health Department of Khorezm Province

Comparative indicators of primary morbidity of mental diseases in cities and districts of Khorezm region for 2022-2023.

Comparative indicators of primary morbidity of mental diseases in cities and districts of Khorezm region for 2022-2023.

(in absolute numbers and per 100,000 inhabitants)

Cities and districts	2022 г		2023 г	
	In absolute figures	Per 100,000 inhabitants bodies	In absolute figures	Per 100,000 live-body
Urgench	52	35,1	58	38,3
Tuprokkala'a	19	33,2	14	23,9
Khiva	29	30,2	33	33,7
Bogotá	60	35,1	52	29,8
Gurlan	43	28,1	52	33,4
Kushkupir	49	27,6	47	26,0
Urgench district	56	27,0	126	59,6
H,azorasp	63	31,4	63	30,9
Honza	53	27,4	57	29,0

Khiva district.	65	43,1	55	35,8
Shovot	62	35,3	43	24,1
Yaigiaritz	45	37,5	27	22,1
Yangibozor	23	25,5	40	43,6
According to regional indicators	**619**	**31,9**	**667**	**33,7**

According to the data of the Health Department of the Khorezm region, the number of of patients with mental illnesses according to general regional indicators in 2023 increased by 48 patients (per 100000 inhabitants) compared to 2022.
2023 increased by 48 patients (per 100,000 inhabitants) compared to 2022.
year

Comparative indicators of primary morbidity of tumour diseases in cities and districts of Khorezm region for 2022-2023

Comparative indicators of primary morbidity of tumour diseases in cities and districts of Khorezm region for 2022-2023.

(in absolute numbers and per 100,000 inhabitants)

Cities and districts	2022 г		2023 г	
	In absolute figures	Per 100,000. residents	In absolute figures	100000 ahzliga
Urgench	139	93,7	147	97,0
Tuprozzal'a	30	52,4	26	44,4
Khiva	89	92,6	89	90,9
Bogotá	106	62,0	114	65,4
Gurlan	93	60,7	92	59,0
Kushkupir	106	59,7	124	68,7
Urgench district	150	72,3	141	66,7
H,azorasp	130	64,9	129	63,2
Honza	193	99,9	185	94,1
Khiva district	92	61,0	96	**62,6**
Shovot	128	72,8	167	93,4
Yangiaritz	89	74,2	76	62,3
Yangibozor	59	65,5	52	56,7
According to regional indicators	**1404**	**72,3**	**1438**	**72,7**

According to the data of the Health Department of the Khorezm region, the number of of patients with oncological diseases according to general regional indicators in 2023 increased by 34 patients (per 100,000 inhabitants) compared to 2022. year

(absolute number and per 100,000 population)

Cities and districts	2022 г		2023 г	
	In absolute figures	Per 100,000. residents	In absolute figures	Per 100,000. residents
Urgench	542	365,4	335	221,1
Tuprokkala'a	131	228,8	101	172,3
Khiva	395	411,0	291	297,2
BOFOT	184	107,6	302	173,2
Gurlan	233	152,1	241	154,6
Kushkupir	419	236,0	289	160,0
Urgench district	384	185,2	513	242,7
Hazorasp	402	200,6	391	191,6
Honka	238	123,1	399	202,9
Khiva district	236	156,4	304	198,1
Shovot	206	117,2	337	188,5
Yangiarik	220	183,5	215	176,2
Yangibozor	130	144,2	136	148,4
According to regional indicators	**3720**	**191,6**	**3854**	**195,0**

According to the data of the Health Department of the Khorezm region, the number of of patients with diabetes mellitus according to general regional indicators in 2023 increased by 134 patients (per 100,000 inhabitants) compared to 2022

Disability in Khorezm region annual information for 2022-2023.

Cities and districts	2022 й			2023 й		
	General	Children	Adults	General	Children	Adults
Urgench	5006	696	4310	5231	727	4504
Tuprokkala'a	1460	276	1184	1577	283	1294
Khiva	3035	458	2577	3225	486	2739
BOFOT	3760	785	2975	4088	838	3250
Gurlan	2990	592	2398	3162	594	2568
Kushkupir	4938	934	4004	5245	969	4276
Urgench district	4926	918	4008	5415	981	4434
Hazorasp	6199	860	5339	6681	889	5792
Honka	4706	906	3800	5017	888	4129
Khiva district	4584	802	3782	5055	820	4235
Shovot	4650	999	3651	5001	1026	3975
Yangiarik	3416	736	2680	3705	783	2922
Yangibozor	2096	434	1662	2254	451	1803
According to regional indicators	**51766**	**9396**	**42370**	**55656**	**9735**	**45921**

According to the data of the Health Department of Khorezm region on general regional indicators disability increased by 3,890 new registered cases in 2023 (per 100,000 inhabitants) compared to 2022

LITERATURE USED

Abdullaev R.B. et al. Impact of environmental problems on the health of the population of Khorezm region. IIMSI ZHARCHYSY. Bulletin of NIMSI. Scientific and informational journal. Kyrgyzstan . Jalal-Abad. 2022. № 2(4). 17-23 p. **Abdullaev R.B.,** Bakhtiyarova **A.M.** Prevalence of digestive system pathology among women of fertile age in the conditions of the Southern Aral Sea region. Collection of scientific papers of the International Scientific and Practical Conference "Role of innovation in medicine". 2024. Urgench. 407 pp.

Abdullaev R.B. et al. Aral crisis: problems of ecological culture and health. // Monograph. Urgench. 2012.-C.120.

Abdullaev R.B., Yakubova A.B. Occurrence of digestive system morbidity in women of reproductive age living in Khorezm Viloyat // Journal of Hepato-Gastroenterological Research. - 2020. - T. 1. - №. 1.

Alibekov L., Nishonov S. Orol fozheasining okibatlari // Fan va turmush. - 1994. - №3. -C. 8-9.

Asadov D.A. Medical and social aspects of maternal mortality in a region with high fertility //Med. zhurn. of Uzbekistan. 1992, №11-12. C.69.

Abdullaev R.B., Hodjaev Sh.A., Ruzmetova M.S. Prevalence of extragenital diseases in women of fertile age living in conditions of ecological disadvantage // Medical Journal of Uzbekistan - 2000.- № 4.-S. 65-67.

Abdullaev R.B. Perebtvirazkova! khvorabisi lunka! twelve-palo! tutyun "us" //V!snik naukoikh dosliženi.-Ukraine.-2000. -№3. -C. 38-39.

Berdimuratova A. Ecological crisis in Priaralie and problems of its solution //Economics and Statics.- 1997. -№11-12. -C. 70-71.

Baltabaev A.A. Prevalence of heart defects in women of childbearing age. //Med.zhurn.uzbekistan 1996. №3. C.29-30.

Hygienic and ecological problems of the hydrosphere and public health in the zone of the Kazakhstan part of the Aral **Sea region /Kulmanov M.E., Amrin K.R., Kenesariev K.I.** and others. //Health Protection of Kazakhstan. -1993. -№3. -C. 17-20.

Bekchanova Y.H. Clinical and pharmacological analysis of hepatoprotectors used for treatment of liver cirrhosis in Khorezm region. Avtoref.diss...d. in medical sciences. Tashkent, 2022. - 60 pp.

Babadjanova F.R.Peculiarities of myocardial adaptation in congenital heart disease in children living in the Aral Sea zone. Tashkent, 2022. - 73 pp.

Goldstein R. Our geoecology //Economics and Statistics. -1996. -№3. -C.6364.

Duschanov B.A. Zhanubiy Orol Buyi minntakasidagi ecologik nokulai vaziyat / Mat.Resp. -1999. - C.2-3.

Iskandarov Sh.T. Evaluation of the effectiveness of new methods of disinfection of drinking and waste water for the prevention of intestinal infections. //Infection, immunity and pharmacology. 1999. № 1 C. 75-77.

Ignatieva N.O., Runkov S.I. Ecological and socio-economic problems of the Aral Sea. // Ogaryov-Online. Mordova. 2023. №4(189). 1-6 pp.

Karimov I.A. Uzbekistan on the threshold of XX century. T. "Uzbekistan". -1997. - C.105128.

Kadirova X. Ecological situation and health of the population of Kazakhstan /Health of Kazakhstan. -1993. -№6. -C. 12-14.

Kazakova R. Ecological situation and human health //Economics and Statistics. - 1997. -№3. -C. 59.

Kosimov E.Y. et al. Tugish yoshidagi hotin-kizlar va homilador ayollarda extragenital kasalliklarning tarkalishi, tashkhisi va sogmlashtirish masa-lalari. //Med.zhurn. of Uzbekistan. 1995. №3. C. 3-6.

Kobilov E. E. et al. Peculiarities of the course of diseases among the population of the southern Aral Sea region // A43 Actual problems of ecology and nature use. - 2021. - T. 22. - C. 307.

Nuraliev N-A. Features of the immune system and microbiocenosis of the large intestine in healthy and diarrhoeal diseases children, living on the territory of the country

In the Southern Priaralie and new approaches to their correction. -Autoref. dissertation for the academic degree of doctor of medical sciences. -Tashkent-2001. - 32 pp.

Navruzov D.K. Age peculiarities of anthropometric indices of different parts of the vertebral column in adolescent children living in the Southern Priaralie. Avtoref. dissertation...Dr.-Ph.D. in medical sciences. Tashkent, 2023. - 102 pp.

Razzakov R.M. Ecological problems of the Aral Sea region /Autoref. dissertation...dr. of geography. sciences. Tashkent, 1997. - 89 pp.

Tileukulova G.S. Impact of the Aral crisis on the countries of Central Asia. // Achievements of science and education. Kazakhstan. 2022. №2(82). 14-16 pp.

Yuldashev O.S. Features of thyroid gland dysfunction and mastopathies in women of fertile age in the Southern Aral Sea region. Tashkent, 2022. - 89 pp

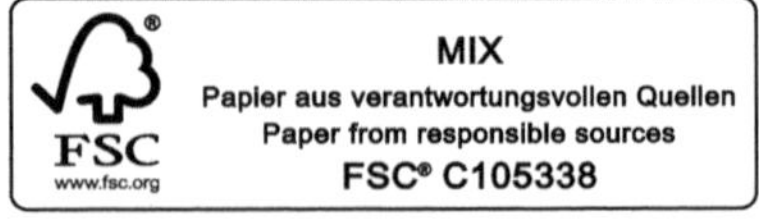

Printed by Books on Demand GmbH, Norderstedt / Germany